Our Unsystematic Healthcare System

Fifth Edition

Grace Budrys

ROWMAN & LITTLEFIELD
Lanham • Boulder • New York • London

Senior Acquisitions Editor: Alyssa Palazzo
Assistant Acquisitions Editor: Samantha Delwarte
Sales and Marketing Inquiries: textbooks@rowman.com

Credits and acknowledgments for material borrowed from other sources, and reproduced with permission, appear on the appropriate pages within the text.

Published by Rowman & Littlefield
An imprint of The Rowman & Littlefield Publishing Group, Inc.
4501 Forbes Boulevard, Suite 200, Lanham, Maryland 20706
www.rowman.com

86-90 Paul Street, London EC2A 4NE

British Library Cataloguing in Publication Information Available

Library of Congress Cataloging-in-Publication Data

Names: Budrys, Grace, 1943– author.
Title: Our unsystematic healthcare system / Grace Budrys.
Description: Fifth edition. | Lanham : Rowman & Littlefield, [2024] | Includes
   bibliographical references and index.
Identifiers: LCCN 2023020013 (print) | LCCN 2023020014 (ebook) | ISBN
   9781538177037 (cloth ; alk. paper) | ISBN 9781538177044 (paperback ; alk. paper) |
   ISBN 9781538177051 (epub)
Subjects: MESH: Delivery of Health Care | Health Policy | Health Care Reform |
   Insurance, Health | United States
Classification: LCC RA418 (print) | LCC RA418 (ebook) | NLM W 84 AA1 | DDC
   362.1—dc23/eng/20230714
LC record available at https://lccn.loc.gov/2023020013
LC ebook record available at https://lccn.loc.gov/2023020014

Contents

Preface

The US healthcare system is a work in progress. It has undergone extensive change since the last edition of this book appeared in 2015. That edition concentrated on the ground-breaking changes introduced by the Affordable Care Act, passed in 2010 and implemented in 2014. This edition is, to some extent, shaped by the unprecedented crisis caused by the onset of the Covid-19 epidemic.

As everyone would undoubtedly agree, public health efforts designed to prevent the spread of Covid-19 did not go smoothly. They quickly became controversial in our highly polarized society. Other events, with health sector implications, added to the polarization. One of the most contentious was the Supreme Court's decision to overturn *Roe v. Wade*, causing social and political turmoil that has not abated. Healthcare providers continue to be confused about interpretation of the law governing abortion in their respective states. There was also the aggressive public health stance the White House took in reaction to the mpox epidemic. It would surely have been far more controversial but did not rise to that level because the surge in cases ended so quickly. This book includes a new chapter on public health in which these issues are discussed after the chapter's primary purpose outlining public health origins, workings, and achievements is fulfilled.

All the chapters in the book have undergone revision, starting with the first chapter. The book begins by posing the question of why the US population does not live as long as people in other countries, even though we spend so much more on health care than they do. I come back to that question in the final chapters of the book.

Chapters on health insurance, health occupations, and hospitals have been updated. We kept hearing how the number of very sick Covid patients overwhelmed health workers and hospitals. Most people are not aware that physicians have become increasingly frustrated by changes in how they are reimbursed. The formula's complexity is pretty amazing. The chapter dealing with hospitals reveals how consolidated they have become, resulting in a declining number of hospital networks that are now enormous. The chapter dealing with the *private health insurance* sector documents steadily increasing vertical and horizontal integration as well, that is, consolidation. The book points to a new development health policy experts warn about—that private equity investment in consolidated physician and hospital networks poses a serious threat to our healthcare arrangements.

The chapter on *public health insurance* focuses on the unprecedented steps the federal government took to avert an increase in uninsurance as people lost their health insurance along with their jobs when Covid caused businesses to close.

I have added a new chapter on the pharmaceutical industry to explore why it is the most reviled participant in our healthcare system. The chapter on other countries considers updated data on life expectancy and national expenditures with consideration of why the United States comes out so poorly on these measures.

The book ends with a new chapter on the social determinants of health. I have added this chapter in response to the concerted effort to convince us that our health depends on personal choices, including how much we eat, exercise, sleep, and so on. The chapter explores the World Health Organization's view that neither behavior nor healthcare arrangements are primarily responsible for people's health. I expand on this position by presenting the American Public Health Association's devastating assessment of what accounts for the health status of individuals and of society as a whole.

I want to thank reviewers who provided helpful suggestions for revision, including Robert Tokle of Idaho State University, Richard Dozal-Lockwood of Portland State University, and Marta Rodriquez-Galan of St. John Fisher University. I am especially grateful for the support I received from Alyssa Palazzo, acquisitions editor at Rowman & Littlefield, and Samantha Delwarte, assistant acquisitions editor, and all the other members of the team. Their patience and practical advice made the work involved in writing this book much more enjoyable.

Chapter 1

Introduction

People in this country don't agree about very much, but they do agree about one thing—health care is too expensive. Drug prices are at the top of the list of complaints. Dramatic personal accounts of the devastating effects of surprise hospital bills appear regularly in the news, helping to reinforce the idea that health care is too expensive. And for those who pay attention to such things, Congress keeps passing new legislation purportedly designed to control healthcare costs. But costs keep going up.

The news media is ready to hold one set of villains after another responsible for rising costs connected to all sorts of healthcare companies. Some end up being found guilty of fraud and are punished; most are not. Punishment generally takes the form of a fine, which, in many cases, looks gigantic to most folks. Healthcare system critics react by saying the organizations build the cost of such penalties into their business plans. Nothing seems to change. It looks like no one knows what to do about the situation. Besides, we can't agree on who we think should be doing it.

I have to admit I miss the on-the-street interviews that occurred during the years just before the Affordable Care Act (ACA), or Obamacare, was legislated over a dozen years ago. People were ready to express strong feelings about the new law. We heard the interviewees saying things like—"I want the government to keep its hands off of my Medicare" or "the Affordable Care Act is better than Obamacare." It was entertaining to listen to for anyone who knew anything about the pending legislation. It revealed how little people knew about the country's healthcare system; or, as a less sanguine interpretation would have it, the extent to which they had been misled about it. There is good reason to believe that is just as true now as it was then.

Curiously, those who complain about the system in one breath are often ready to proclaim that the US healthcare system is the best in the world in the next breath. They are eager to point out that people in other countries have long waits for doctors' appointments and inordinate delays in having surgery. Not only that, they say, but look at all the people who come to the

1

United States to get health care because, they happily assert, our technological capabilities, medications, and doctors are all superior to those available in other countries.

The question of whether the United States has more high-tech medical capabilities than other countries is easy to answer. The Organisation for Economic Co-operation and Development (OECD) provides us with a comparison of the number of computerized tomography (CT) scanners and magnetic resonance imagery (MRI) machines across its thirty-eight member countries, the most economically developed countries in the world. Let's compare our med-tech capacity to that of countries to which we often compare ourselves.

As table 1.1 makes clear, other countries have the same kinds of high-tech medical diagnostic equipment, and in some cases, they have more than we do. It is also worth mentioning that the United States isn't alone in manufacturing high-tech machines. The machines are manufactured all over the world by companies that are globally owned. And we can't even be credited for inventing them all. CT scanners were invented in England.

Then there's the question of whether having more high-tech medical machinery translates into better health. The indicator used to indicate health status across populations is life expectancy. Let's look at who lives longest. Table 1.2 reports life expectancy as of 2019, starting with countries with the longest life expectancy, according to the World Bank, which bases its numbers on World Health Organization (WHO) data collected in 219 countries. I have left out countries on that list that can boast even longer life expectancy but to which we do not compare ourselves because they are very small, such as Hong Kong, Macau, and Singapore.

Table 1.1. CT and MRI machines per one million population, 2017

Country	CT*	Country	MRI**
1. Japan	111	1. Japan	57
2. United States	43	2. United States	38
3. Switzerland	40	3. Germany	35
4. Italy	40	4. Italy	34
5. Germany	35	5. Switzerland	27
6. Spain	20	6. Spain	18
7. France	19	7. France	16
8. Canada	15	8. Canada	10
9. United Kingdom	10	9. United Kingdom	9

*OECD. "Computed Tomography (CT) Scanners." https://data.oecd.org/healtheqt/computed-tomography-ct-scanners.htm#indicator-chart.

**OECD. "Magnetic Resonance Imaging (MRI) Units." https://data.oecd.org/healtheqt/magnetic-resonance-imaging-mri-units.htm.

Table 1.2. Life expectancy in 2019

Country	Life Expectancy
1. Japan	84.8
2. Switzerland	84.3
3. Italy	84.1
4. Spain	83.9
5. Australia	83.6
6. Sweden	83.5
7. Norway	83.4
8. France	83.2
9. Canada	82.8
10. United States	78.2

Source: World Bank. "Life Expectancy at Birth, Total (years)." United Nations Population Division, World Population Prospects, 2022 Review. https://data.worldbank.org/indicator/SP.DYN.LE00.IN.

So, what do you think—would you conclude there is a close relationship between the number of high-tech machines a country has and life expectancy? It doesn't look like there is, does it?

How about the amount of money a country devotes to health care? Is it possible that other countries are ready to spend more on providing health care for their populations, and that is what accounts for longer life expectancy? The measure used to calculate national expenditures on health care is the percent of the gross domestic product (GDP). (Think of GDP as a pie chart representing every dollar that changes hands in the country—covering consumption, imports and exports, and government spending, with health care as a slice.) The data in table 1.3 come from the World Bank based on statistics collected by the WHO.

The interpretation of the data we have just considered is not complicated. We can see that the United States spends a far greater proportion of its GDP on health care than other countries; we have a shorter life expectancy, and it doesn't look like having as much high-tech equipment as we have is providing us with better health.

Before we leave this topic, it is essential to note an important fact not captured by these tables. All the countries to which we compare ourselves provide health insurance for their entire population—they have *universal coverage*. Indeed, virtually all economically advanced countries manage to do so. We do not.

It seems to me that one can only conclude that many other countries must be doing something right to bring about longer life expectancy.[1] Is there anything we can learn from them? Maybe a better question is the following: Is there anything we are willing to learn from them? Apparently not, given that the data we are looking at are readily available to anyone who might be interested. The data don't seem to be making much of an impression on folks who

Table 1.3. Life expectancy compared to percent of GDP expenditure on health, 2019

Country	Life Expectancy*	GDP**
1. Japan	84.8	10.7
2. Switzerland	84.3	11.3
3. Italy	84.1	8.7
4. Spain	83.9	9.1
5. Australia	83.6	9.9
6. Sweden	83.5	10.9
7. Norway	83.4	10.5
8. France	83.2	11.1
9. Canada	82.8	10.8
10. United States	78.2	16.8

* World Bank. 2022 Review.

** World Bank. 2022. "Current Health Expenditure (%GDP)." World Health Organization, Global Health Database. Accessed January 20, 2022. https://data.worldbank.org/indicator/SH.XPD.CHEX.GD.ZS.

oppose making the kinds of changes in this country's healthcare arrangements that might lead to better health outcomes and longer life expectancy. But let's not give up. If more people come to understand how the health system works, there's a greater chance more people will be ready to press for positive changes that will benefit us all. The discussion presented in the chapters to follow aims to promote that goal.

This book has four ambitious objectives: first, to describe the organizational structure of the US healthcare system; second, to provide an account of its origins; third, to assess how well it serves us; and finally, to consider factors responsible for the population's health status that operate outside of our healthcare system.

Because we have just lived through, and continue to deal with, something the world has not confronted for over a hundred years, a global pandemic, Covid-19 is unavoidably a big part of the story. That is, in fact, the subject of the next chapter. The Covid epidemic had an enormous impact on society as a whole and the healthcare system in particular. Now that the crisis is over, health policy analysts are urging healthcare organizations and institutions to be prepared for the next epidemic, which they assure us is inevitable. Whether we are better prepared remains to be seen.

Chapter 3 focuses on health insurance offered by private companies. Chapter 4 turns to public health insurance, that is, health insurance provided by the government. Chapter 5 discusses health occupations. Chapter 6 focuses on hospitals. Chapter 7 examines how the pharmaceutical industry works. Chapter 8 expands on the discussion presented in this chapter by offering a more comprehensive assessment of the healthcare systems in other countries. The final chapter, chapter 9, is where we explore factors that affect health status outside of what the healthcare system is designed to address—the "social determinants of health."

I should add that you are about to confront a rapidly shifting scenario. Not only do statistics on such basic facts as life expectancy, health outcomes, and expenditures change from one year to the next, meaning what is written here might be outdated by the time you read it, but interpretations also change as more research is conducted to explore the reasons behind the changes. Additionally, the political arena, where laws governing healthcare arrangements are crafted, has been particularly active over the last few years.

However, once you finish the book, you will have a good sense of virtually all the factors that affect the health status of individuals in this country, so you won't be surprised when someone brings any of them up. You will certainly have a much better understanding of how the health system works and its relationship to people's health than the vast majority of folks in this country, many who hold strong views about it all but don't have a firm grasp of the facts. I encourage you to spread the word.

Chapter 2

Public Health

The public health sector's contribution to society's welfare was not something to which people in this country were paying much attention—until Covid-19 came on the scene at the beginning of 2020. That's when anyone who tuned in to the news couldn't help but discover what public health is all about. We were suddenly hearing from one public health expert after another in what seemed like a never-ending loop of media presentations. Biomedical researchers explained why the Covid-19 virus was so contagious. They did it graphically, providing us with what became the popular depiction of the virus—a red, round ball full of spikes, each capable of transferring the virus. Epidemiologists explained how it was being transmitted. They said it was airborne, being spread through the air with each breath a person expels, as opposed to contact with infected objects. Biostatisticians presented charts tracking the number of people diagnosed with the disease and reporting it as the morbidity rate, going to report the number dying from the disease (i.e., the mortality rate). Social and behavioral scientists connected to public health agencies, schools of public health, and other health-oriented research centers offered analyses of the data. They identified regions of the country where the virus was spreading faster than in other places. They explained who was most susceptible, namely, the elderly and those with suppressed immune systems.

Public health policy analysts who focus on international issues told us that the Covid-19 virus was spreading in countries worldwide, meaning it was a global pandemic requiring action from the federal government. But President Donald Trump and his followers dismissed what the experts had to say, claiming that the virus was no more serious than the flu. Meanwhile, the mortality rate just kept rising.

Public health organizations at all levels began calling for the use of masks. Government organizations, joined by many in the private sector, started requiring people to wear masks at various venues and settings. While this caused some people to search for the most efficient masks, it inspired others to reject advice on masking, claiming the masking requirement was a government infringement on personal liberty.

By the end of 2020, two versions of a vaccine were introduced in what everyone recognized to be an amazingly short period of time. The offer of funding from the Trump administration helped facilitate that. Pharmaceutical companies were eager to respond to the promise of vast numbers of customers worldwide. The Operation Warp Speed legislation of 2021 temporarily authorized vaccine production before it was officially approved in response to the public health emergency. (We'll return to the pharmaceutical sector and its performance in chapter 7.) Home testing kits appeared not long after that. The federal government made the kits and vaccines available to everyone at no cost. Booster shots came shortly after that.

The vaccines proved to be highly effective. While people continued to be infected after being vaccinated, far fewer required hospitalization. The death rate began to drop. The epidemic began to recede. Hospitals and hospital workers were no longer overwhelmed; the economy started to recover as people stopped isolating themselves; students started returning to in-class learning. In other words, by the spring of 2022, things started to return to normal, a different normal, but no longer at the crisis stage. This is when experts stopped seeing Covid-19 as a pandemic and began treating it as endemic, something that we will be forced to accept as a continuing risk and likely require an annual vaccine to fight off infection.

As of this writing, it's been three years since we first encountered Covid-19. In reviewing its trajectory, virologists are ready to report that it took six months for the initial mutation to appear, but after that, it took only six weeks for each new iteration. By the middle of 2022, seventy known mutations had come into existence since Covid-19 first appeared. The experts say this is roughly what they would have predicted. Many more strains are thought to have slipped through without being identified. And more keep appearing. Although there was no assurance it would turn out this way, the latest variants are far more infectious but less lethal.

Why review what everybody already knows about the country's experience with Covid-19? Because it illustrates how public health works and the challenges it faces.

PUBLIC HEALTH AND CONTROVERSY

At one level, what the public health establishment aims to accomplish is very simple—prevent the onset of illness and disease. At another level, that objective is very complicated because there is no single clear approach for achieving that objective and no scientific discipline that indicates how to accomplish it. The upshot is that practitioners with training in various disciplines, such as those just mentioned, have been working together to provide assessments, create diagnostic tools, and identify treatment strategies.

One way, an oversimplified way, of looking at how public health operates is to contrast it to the work doctors do. Doctors treat individual patients. The "patient" public health practitioners treat is the community. That's a big difference. But how the two approach their respective patients is comparable. Public health practitioners, like doctors, start by assessing the health of the population, diagnosing the problem, working on identifying the cause of the patient's problem, and, finally, devising a strategy to treat the patient's problem. A major difference between what doctors do and what public health practitioners do is that the former largely focus on a cure after patients become sick, and the latter focus on preventing patients from becoming sick in the first place.

One would think most people would see the effort to prevent illness and disease as laudable and have no reason to find fault. Yet, opposition is ever-present. Public health assessments, diagnoses, and treatment strategies are treated as controversial for at least four reasons.[1]

To begin with, there are economic implications. Companies making products that have a direct negative impact on health, such as cigarette companies, companies producing opioids, and gun manufacturers, for example, have vigorously objected to public health assessments documenting damaging health effects. Corporations that pollute the air or water are quick to argue that the public health environmental assessments are wrong. A long list of industries that rely on coal and petroleum products strongly oppose such assessments, including companies producing steel, fertilizer, cosmetics, and plastics, to name a few. Those who invest in these companies can be counted on to oppose legislation calling for changes to make a product safer because introducing safety measures is sure to cut into financial returns.

Another source of controversy is the claim that public health efforts infringe on individual liberty. As we can all agree, this argument was front and center with regard to masking and vaccination. Why masks became so controversial is not entirely clear. For lack of a better explanation, I'll leave it at that it has something to do with the times we live in. (A topic we will return to in chapter 9.) After all, the prohibition against smoking in public places was embraced without a huge fight. Drunk driving declined in response to public health campaigns. Similarly, one doesn't hear too many people objecting to seat belts anymore. Prior to the onset of Covid, opposition to the requirement that children be vaccinated before entering school was thought to be something embraced by small numbers of people associated with fringe groups. That has changed.

Religious and moral opposition is a third source of controversy. Resistance to public health recommendations is easier to explain in some instances than others. Matters related to sex are especially likely to arouse opposition. This includes sex education and the availability of contraceptive products. Needle exchanges inspire moral outrage on the part of some who may not be religious. Religious opposition was most prominently displayed as some churches not only rejected masking but flaunted the mandate meant to avoid indoor crowding. Public health practitioners warned that such gatherings were likely "super-spreader" events.

Finally, there is the specter of political controversy. It is not unusual to find politicians ready to oppose inconvenient public health assessments, diagnoses, and treatment recommendations to which some of their constituents objected. This is especially likely when politicians find that those constituents are ready to back up their preferences with funding or assurance that they can deliver the vote.

Representatives of the public health community find it difficult to match the passion of dedicated opponents. Presentation of scientific findings doesn't offer the kind of spectacle that opponents with strong but ungrounded beliefs are ready to employ. Let's face it, dealing in facts is just not as sexy as spinning the exciting, creative tales that those who oppose science can come up with.

PUBLIC HEALTH ORIGINS AND DEVELOPMENT

Discussion about the origins of public health invariably starts with the story of Dr. John Snow and the Broad Street pump. Snow identified a particular London water pump as the source of the spread of cholera. It took some effort to convince people that what he said was true. At the time, in 1853, people were convinced that cholera was spread through a "miasma." However, the statistics Snow presented were indisputable. His calculations indicated that people who got their water from the Broad Street pump were getting cholera at a far greater rate than those who got their water from one of the other two other pumps in the area. He is credited with being the father of epidemiology.

The United States has its own hero, Samuel Shattuck, recognized as the father of public health. He gained this acclaim for his 1850 report on the "sanitary survey of the State" of Massachusetts. The report led to a model state public law passed in 1866, which was emulated by states across the country.

The origins of public health as an institution can be traced to a much earlier date. The history of the public health enterprise in the United States is not well known, probably because it is so convoluted. I expect you will agree when you consider the account that follows.

The story begins with the Act for the Relief of Sick and Disabled Seaman passed in 1798. The work of dealing with sick seamen led to the creation of the Marine Hospital Service in 1870. This operation was reorganized into the US Public Health Service Commercial Corps in 1889. It was renamed the Public Health Marine Service in 1912. It became the US Public Health Service (PHS) in 1944. It went through a number of additional organizational shuffles after that, settling into its present status in 1987. The PHS currently employs 6,500 commissioned officers who answer to the Surgeon General. The Surgeon General reports to the Office of the Assistant Secretary of Health (OASH), who reports, in turn, to the director of the Department of Health and Human Services (HHS). In other words, the PHS is a subunit of a much larger institution. At the same time, public health is a vast enterprise that functions at the federal, state, and local level and through a wide range of government agencies as well as nongovernmental organizations. For now, let's focus on public health as a federal government enterprise.

As just mentioned, the PHS stands under the HHS umbrella. The HHS is a cabinet-level organization; that is, it answers directly to the President of the United States. HHS encompasses nine public health agencies.[2] HHS oversees ten regional offices, numerous advisory committees, task forces, and special initiatives. This organization came into existence in 1980 when Education was split off from what was then the US Department of Health, Education and Welfare (HEW).

So how did the original PHS end up being a division of HHS? As I said, this is a convoluted story.

The explanation is that agencies dedicated to one health issue or another kept growing out of work being carried out by the PHS. The National Institutes of Health (NIH), created in 1887, provides a good example. It grew out of the Laboratory of Hygiene, which was sponsored by the PHS to conduct research aimed at controlling the spread of cholera. The Laboratory of Hygiene turned into the National Institute of Health (NIH) (*singular*) in 1937. It was renamed the National Institutes of Health (NIH) (*plural*) in recognition of the ever-increasing number of agencies coming into existence to deal with specific illnesses under the auspices of this agency in 1948.

The Centers for Disease Control and Prevention (CDC), one of the eight units under the Department of Health and Human Services dedicated to health as opposed to human services, was established in 1946. It grew out of the Communicable Diseases Center, a small operation in Atlanta, Georgia, that was focused on controlling the spread of malaria. The Communicable Diseases Center expanded early in its existence, adding an internal unit called the Epidemic Intelligence Center to track common health threats. The workers associated with this Center were known as "disease detectives." The Communicable Diseases Center did not receive much support and may not have survived if it were not for two waves of illness that occurred in the 1950s that it helped to end: (1) polio and (2) a massive influenza epidemic. It became the CDC in 1970.

The Federal Drug Administration (FDA), another agency under the HHS umbrella, traces its roots to eleven doctors who, in 1820, created the US Pharmacopeia Record, which was basically a list of standard drugs. The American Medical Association (AMA) assisted in this effort by establishing a voluntary drug approval arrangement in 1905. This encouraged the government to pass the Food and Drug Act in 1906 to establish drug safety; it did not require evidence of drug efficacy then. The FDA faced a steady stream of opposition from drug makers until 1962 when its future was suddenly no longer in doubt. This was the result of the Thalidomide crisis when an officer associated with the FDA worked to prevent approval of Thalidomide, a sleeping pill used by pregnant women that caused thousands of European children to be born with serious physical defects. The public credited the agency for this invaluable decision. It also allowed the passage of legislation that required—for the first time—drug makers to prove drug efficacy.

As an aside, it is interesting to note the role the Supreme Court has played over the years in ruling against the work being carried out by agencies dedicated to public health. To illustrate, it rejected the FDA's claim that cigarettes were "drug delivery devices" in 1995 and, in 2000, ruled that the FDA did not have the authority to regulate tobacco as a drug. The position taken by the Supreme Court in opposition to public health agency efforts to protect public health was reaffirmed in 2022 when it ruled that the Environmental Protection Agency (EPA) does not have the authority to limit carbon emissions in the interest of protecting clean air and combating climate change. And in the same year, it overturned the constitutional right to an abortion established in the *Roe v. Wade* case, which caused a national outcry on the part of those who maintain abortion is essential to public health. More on this decision later in this chapter.

The Health Resources and Services Administration (HRSA) came into existence in 1973. It replaced the Bureau of Health Services, established in 1966 upon the closure of the Bureau of Medical Services, and the Bureau of State Services, created earlier in 1945. Other agencies under the auspices of HHS include the just-mentioned EPA; the Agency for Health Research and Quality (AHRQ); the Agency for Toxic Substance and Disease Registry (ATSDR); Indian Health Service (IHS); and the Substance Abuse and Mental Health Services Administration (SAMHSA).

The stories documenting the creation and development of each of these agencies are all attention-grabbing. They include accounts of the hurdles the agencies had to overcome to be where they are today and lists of achievements they are proud to claim. What is most striking, at least to me, is how unplanned or unsystematic the steps were that led to what these institutions look like today.

It was not until 1976 that Congress determined an organization specifically devoted to public health needed to be established. This is when the Office of Disease Prevention and Health Promotion (ODPHP) was created "to lead disease prevention and health promotion efforts in the United States." It answers to the Office of the Assistant Secretary for Health, which operates under the auspices of HHS. One of this organization's main responsibilities is coordinating the government's main health-focused website—health.gov—and its microsites.

STATE AND LOCAL PUBLIC HEALTH AGENCIES

Every state in the country has its own state public health department. There are roughly 3,000 health departments at the local level. The relationship between the state health department and local health departments varies from state to state. The local departments may be part of the state health department, may be loosely affiliated, or completely independent. Rhode Island, Vermont, and Delaware have a state public health department but no local health departments, while Georgia has 159 local departments.

Most health departments belong to the National Association of County and City Health Officials (NACCHO). The organization was established as the National Association of County Health Officials in 1965 and renamed in 1994.

NACCHO lists six objectives in outlining the work that public health departments under its auspices are expected to perform.[3] The first objective is enough to make clear how challenging the task is that health departments set forth for themselves.

1. Track and investigate health problems and hazards in the community; analyze data to determine risks and problems that drive specific programs related to communicable and chronic diseases; food, water, insect, and other "vector-borne" outbreaks, biological and radiological hazards; and public health disasters.
2. Prepare and respond to public health emergencies.
3. Develop, apply, and enforce policies, laws, and regulations that improve health and ensure safety.
4. Lead efforts to mobilize communities around important health issues.
5. Link people to health services.
6. Achieve excellence in public health practice through a trained workforce, evaluations, and evidence-based programs.

A new organization came on the scene in response to a 2003 Institute of Medicine (IOM) report to make sure that public health departments carry out those tasks.

As an aside, you might be interested to know more about the IOM. We will be referring to reports it has authored throughout the book. It was established in 1970 as an arm of the National Academy of Sciences, chartered under President Abraham Lincoln in 1863. In 2015, the IOM voted to change its name to National Academy of Medicine. It is now part of the National Academies of Science, Engineering and Medicine with 1,900 elected members. Its purpose is to issue reports based on the input of the experts it brings together "to facilitate discussion, discovery, and critical cross-disciplinary thinking." It responds to requests from Congress, government agencies, and organizations. The experts are reimbursed for expenses but receive no compensation.

The upshot of the IOM report was the formation of a National Steering Committee to consider the benefits of accreditation. The Robert Wood Johnson Foundation, with the support of the CDC, convened public health stakeholders to review the matter the following year. That led to the creation of the Public Health Accreditation Board in 2007. The Board released a set of standards for vetting in 2009–2010. The standards were approved, and the accreditation effort was launched in 2011. The Board's 2021 report indicates that over 72 percent of agencies have achieved accreditation.

As of 2015, the Public Health Accreditation Board became home to two new centers: the Public Health National Center for Innovations and the Center for School Health Innovation and Quality. The Public Health National Center for Innovations is currently gathering success stories reported by agencies across the country with the aim of inspiring other organizations. In 2000, in collaboration with the de Beaumont Foundation, it worked to revise the 10 Essential Public Health Services (EPHS) identified in 1994. The new list is meant "to provide a framework for public health to protect and promote the health of *all people in all communities* (sic)."

The EPHS list is published on the CDC website.

1. Monitor health status to identify and solve community health problems
2. Diagnose and investigate health problems and health hazards in the community
3. Inform, educate, and empower people about health issues
4. Mobilize community partnerships and action to identify and solve health problems
5. Develop policies and plans that support individual and community health efforts
6. Enforce laws and regulations that protect health and ensure safety

7. Link people to needed personal services and assure the provision of health care when otherwise unavailable
8. Assure competent public and personal healthcare workforce
9. Evaluate effectiveness, accessibility, and quality of personal and population-based health services
10. Research for new insights and innovative solutions to health problems[4]

The National Public Health Performance Standards (NPHPS), a framework that came into existence in 1998, operates to help "identify areas for system improvement, strengthen state and local partnerships, and ensure that a strong system is in place for providing the 10 essential public health services."

NONGOVERNMENTAL PUBLIC HEALTH

The American Public Health Association is the leading nongovernmental organization representing public health practitioners and researchers. Founded in 1872, it held its first meeting in 1873 and has continued to hold annual meetings since then. It began publishing a scholarly journal, the *American Journal of Public Health*, in 1911 with the mission of advancing public health research, policy, practice, and education.

PUBLIC HEALTH ACCOMPLISHMENTS

Each of the organizations mentioned so far makes its mission clear in the materials it publishes. Each outlines the goals it seeks to accomplish. The goals are all health-related. They are all, without question, enormously ambitious.

Does that make you wonder how well is the public health community doing in attaining those goals? In order to answer this question, it is important to step back and reflect on how the goals are measured.

The Office of Disease Prevention and Health Promotion (ODPHP) has issued a list of goals accompanied by measurable objectives every decade since 1980. This project originated in 1979 with what the ODPHP says was a landmark report entitled *Healthy People: The Surgeon General's Report on Health Promotion and Disease Prevention*. This was followed by the release of the "Healthy People 1990" document in 1980. The two primary objectives it set forth were decreasing deaths throughout the life span and independence among older adults. New Healthy People documents have come out every decade since then, outlining specific objectives, such as reduction of health disparities, access to preventive services, and creation of social and physical environments that promote good health. The "Healthy People 2030" report states that it is building "on knowledge gained over the last 4 decades and has an increased focus on health equity, social determinants of health, and health literacy—with a new focus on well-being."[5]

HHS publishes an assessment at the end of each decade evaluating the degree to which the objectives outlined in the reports were attained. The most recent review states that a key lesson from the Healthy People initiative is that a plan with achievable goals

> can guide individuals, organizations, communities, and other stakeholders to improve health. . . . In addition, we have learned how important it is to monitor progress toward achieving Healthy People objectives and to share high-quality data and feedback. That's why we've used rigorous objective selection criteria and why we've made sure Healthy People 2030 data are timely, easy to find, and easy to use.[6]

That may be, but a closer look makes clear that the objectives set forth in each of the Healthy People reports constitute a monumental challenge. Consider that the original 1990 report specified 358 measurable objectives related to (1) health conditions, (2) health behaviors, (3) populations, (4) systems and settings, and (5) social determinants of health. The number of objectives has expanded greatly since then.

The current final review of what was accomplished with regard to the 2020 Healthy People document indicates that much, but certainly not everything, was accomplished. That all the objectives were not attained should be surprising given how ambitious the initiative was—1,318 objectives, of which 1,111 were measurable. The summary reports on 985 trackable objectives.

34 percent of the targets were met or exceeded
21 percent improved
31 percent saw little or no detectable change
14 percent got worse[7]

The list of targets that were met includes: air quality index, children exposed to secondhand smoke, infant death rate, adults meeting aerobic physical activity and muscle strengthening activity, and adolescent smoking within the past thirty days.

The list of targets that got worse includes the following: injury deaths, suicide, adolescent major depressive episodes over the last twelve months, and obesity.

So how should we interpret these results? Without getting too metaphysical about it, it's worth pointing out that evaluating the success of preventive efforts is problematic. It's much easier to evaluate success or failure when the objective is a concrete task, such as curing a person who has a diagnosed illness for which there is a known treatment. It is much harder to take credit for preventing something from happening, like keeping a person from contracting the disease. After all, maybe the problem would not have occurred without any intervention. That's probably unlikely in most instances. Public health problems aren't about to go away without a concerted effort on the part of dedicated public health workers. Going back to the list of targets that got worse, there is no list of agreed-upon preventive steps that would ensure a drop in injury deaths or suicide deaths. Obesity is a multifactorial problem that requires cooperation on the part of many actors. There is a growing body of evidence that it is due to factors other than diet. But to the extent that diet is an important factor, some politicians are ready to oppose measures that would affect industries that contribute to the prevalence of obesity because the industries contribute to the politicians' campaigns. Reducing adolescent depressive episodes is not something the public health system is equipped to address, certainly not alone and maybe not even in collaboration with a range of other interested parties.

EFFICACY OF THE COVID VACCINE

In a final note on Covid mortality rates, we refer to a study by Harvard researchers, analyzing data across all 435 congressional districts from April 2021 to March 2022. They found that Covid death rates were 11 percent higher in states with Republican-controlled governments and 26 percent higher in areas where voters lean conservative.[8] Another study found that counties at the "10th highest level of Trump votes" had over three times as many deaths as counties in the "10th lowest level of Trump votes."[9] Public health researchers say that using political affiliation to account for variation in mortality introduces a novel but highly predictive variable. How the public health community deals with this observation is not something anyone is prepared to address, at least not to date.

A RECENT SPECIAL CASE

The monkeypox outbreak that started in the spring of 2022 illustrates the challenge the public health community faces—first, some history. The virus was identified in laboratory monkeys in 1958. The first human case was recorded in 1970. An outbreak occurred in Texas in 2003 when people purchased pet prairie dogs that had come into contact with a shipment of diseased animals imported from Ghana. The people who were infected had mild symptoms.

The source of the 2022 outbreak is not clear, but it turned out to be global. The WHO, which was involved in tracking it, announced it wants the virus to be renamed and called "mpox."

Its spread was extremely rapid, with the first cases in the United States identified in April, rising to about 3,600 cases by July. The population at greatest risk was identified as men who had sex with men. While some who became infected had no symptoms, others developed painful sores.

The Biden White House appointed a National Monkeypox Response Coordinator as well as a Deputy Coordinator. It took only a few weeks for public health researchers to find that the virus was closely related to smallpox and that the smallpox vaccine was an effective deterrent. Monkeypox was declared a public health emergency on August 4, which allowed the government to scale up the response with data collection, outreach, and free vaccines. Just as fast as it appeared, mpox began a steep decline within days of that declaration. Public health researchers point to three reasons for its decline but are not sure which is the most important: (1) a change in behavior among men who had sex with many partners; (2) the vaccine; and (3) a build-up of immunity after exposure to the virus.[10] This is not to say the virus has been eliminated. It made its appearance again in June of 2023.

This case shows, for a start, how unpredictable viruses are. It shows that luck can play an unexpected role. There was no need to devote time, effort, and expense to finding a vaccine—an old vaccine (for smallpox) was found to work, and a ready supply was available. It also shows that a rapid political response giving the public health community the tools to identify and respond to the outbreak played a critical role in bringing attention to the threat of the virus and its rapid decline. Deciding whether such an aggressive response is required is not easily determined.

In fact, not long after mpox dropped off the public health radar, a new virus hit the scene. The autumn months of 2022 found large numbers of American children suffering from respiratory syncytial virus (RVS). Adults infected with RVS have mild symptoms, young children are at risk of developing pneumonia, and infants are at risk of death. One of the side effects of the Covid epidemic is that very young children who were isolated to protect them from Covid did not develop immunity to a range of viruses in their daily lives. The risk presented by concurrent viruses, Covid, RVS, and seasonal flu resulted in a new word being added to the social media vocabulary—*tripledemic*. It is also true that this threat to the country's health evaporated over the next few months. That is fortunate because the public health community is limited in what it can do to prevent RVS since there is no vaccine. It can track the number of children who are infected and offer advice on prevention, which is the same as advice on preventing any other respiratory infection.

In short, until there is an antiviral vaccine that covers a wide range of viruses, which is, in fact, in the testing stage right now, the public health community is limited in what it can do in the face of the spread of some viruses. At the same time, defining a viral outbreak as a crisis, whether or not treatment is available, can provide the public health community with the tools to help stop its spread.

ANOTHER RECENT CASE

The upheaval brought on by the 2022 Supreme Court ruling in the *Dobbs v. Jackson Women's Health Organization* case overturning the *Roe v. Wade* decision is another instance in which the public health community sees reason to issue policy statements. Anticipating the ruling, public health researchers sought to establish what services public health departments across the country had been providing to date. They found the following:

> Health departments have been involved with issues related to abortion since the 1970s, particularly with regard to surveillance (e.g., [sic] tracking the number and characteristics of women obtaining abortions, types of procedures, and service locations), clinical quality improvements, and conducting research syntheses. These roles have expanded over time, most notably in the past decade. Recent legislation has required governmental health agencies to take on new roles in relation to abortion, including developing content for state-mandated structural standards.[11]

While the ruling did not come as a surprise, neither the public health community nor the country as a whole was prepared to deal with the implications. Right-to-life advocates celebrated the court ruling, but even they were not prepared. It took only a few days for differences of opinion in their ranks about exceptions for incest, rape, and the life of the mother to erupt. At the same time, those opposed to the decision adopted a new label for the abortion ban, calling it "forced birth." Women from all walks of life who had had abortions went public about their experiences. Some talked about the socioeconomic barriers that led them to choose abortion. Others talked about life-threatening conditions that caused them to abort and, in some cases, abort a wanted pregnancy.

The Biden administration reacted to the Supreme Court decision with an executive order directing HHS and other federal agencies to identify actions to protect access to the full range of reproductive healthcare services, including contraception and abortion.

The fact that the Supreme Court left regulation of abortion up to states is responsible for much of the turmoil. At least sixteen state governments immediately announced that they would impose restrictions. Two weeks later, the citizens in a politically conservative state, Kansas, voted overwhelmingly to oppose their state government's attempt to ban abortion. Other state governments planning to impose restrictions readied themselves to face state court challenges. The challenges are timely, given that January of 2023 marks the fiftieth anniversary of the *Roe v. Wade* decision.

Twenty-one states have instituted lawsuits challenging abortion bans as of this date.[12] They fall into three categories: (1) constitutional challenges focusing on liberty, due process, and privacy; (2) healthcare amendment challenges based on state constitutions that include the right to make healthcare decisions; and (3) religious freedom challenges charging that abortion bans infringe on the religious rights and beliefs of people who do not subscribe to what they say is the underlying Christian doctrine. A lawsuit in Florida launched by a Florida synagogue charges discrimination since, in its belief system, life begins only after a person is born.

The *Roe v. Wade* decision provoked responses from a range of organizations. Those representing doctors, nurses, and hospitals expressed outrage, taking the position that abortion is a medical matter, not something to be decided by politicians or lawyers. Emergency room doctors and hospital emergency room department heads found themselves in a tough situation. The Supreme Court decision conflicts with the Emergency Medical Treatment and Labor Act (EMTALA), in effect since 1987. EMTALA requires emergency physicians and hospitals to 1) screen all patients coming to the ER regardless of their ability to pay, 2) stabilize the patient, and 3) transfer the patient, if necessary, only after the patient is stabilized. The medical community maintains that if an abortion is required to "stabilize" the patient, then the doctors are obligated to perform the procedure. However, medical practitioners continue to fear the consequences of breaking the law. The question is—which law? While the Supreme Court left abortion restrictions to the states, federal law takes precedence over state law. How this is settled remains to be seen.

Quite a few major corporations reacted to the Supreme Court ruling by announcing they would stop expanding their businesses in states that restrict abortion. Some offered to cover the costs of employee relocation to a state that does not restrict abortion. Other companies announced readiness to cover employees' travel expenses to obtain an abortion. An unknown number of companies debating how to respond indicated they were counting on their insurance carriers to deal with the problem. Insurance companies are required to cover medically necessary pregnancy care as outlined in the Pregnancy

Discrimination Act of 1978, that is, to cover high-risk pregnancies which could reasonably require an abortion to save the life of the woman. This law has not been challenged to date. Then there are other laws that might present more problems. For example, it is not clear how companies promising to cover travel expenses of employees seeking an abortion in another state would respond if they were charged with discrimination by persons seeking to travel to obtain a variety of other treatments under the Mental Health Parity and Addiction Equity Act. All of this is unexplored legal territory.

One piece of legislation has received considerable public attention, Texas Senate Bill 8, referred to as the "vigilante abortion law." It offers a $10,000 bounty to anyone reporting a person helping a woman obtain an abortion while fining the helper that amount. It lost its first court battle. One problem with the law is that it does not make clear what "help" might entail. A question raised by one commentator may or may not be tongue-in-cheek: Can a librarian be reported for helping someone search for information on abortion providers?

What about medications that bring about abortion? In January of 2023, the FDA announced that such medications could be distributed by drug stores even as some politicians propose banning them, a matter likely to be disputed in court by some states.

A different set of problems associated with health insurance has to do with the Hyde Amendment. It restricts insurance company policies sold through state health insurance marketplaces from covering abortion. Medicaid, the Children's Health Insurance Program, and Medicare are also prohibited from covering abortion expenses. States may, however, use their own funds for that purpose. Seven states do so: California, Illinois, Maine, Maryland, New York, Oregon, and Washington. The Hyde Amendment also affects other government health programs over which states have no authority, including the Veterans Administration, the military, federal prisons, and the Federal Employee Health Benefits Program.

The effort to restrict abortion raises another concern for those who focus on health disparities. It is generally assumed that women who can afford to travel to another state will be able to obtain an abortion regardless of the Supreme Court ruling. Poor women may not be able to do so. Because more people of color and Indigenous people are poor, they are the ones who will find it hard to obtain an abortion. More than half the abortions in 2019 were among women of color. The abortion rate per 1,000 was 23.8 for black women, 11.7 among Hispanic women, and 6.6 among white women.[13] Women of color are at risk of higher pregnancy-related mortality rates due to socioeconomic and racial inequality. The inability to obtain an abortion when faced with life-threatening pregnancy complications promises to increase the rate of maternal mortality among women of color.

The Supreme Court ruling has given rise to discussion of a wide range of implications, for example, the societal impact of "forced births" that result in an unwanted child. A fact being raised by some is that the introduction of legal abortion in 1973, resulting from the *Roe v. Wade* decision, coincides with a significant drop in homicide rates during the decade of the 1990s.[14] No one is prepared to say this is the primary reason behind the drop in homicide rates. However, there is reason to believe it is a contributing factor.

Finally, some observers express concern that the Supreme Court ruling embraces a position not shared by the majority of Americans. According to the Pew Research Center, 62 percent of people in this country disapprove of the Supreme Court's decision.[15] Further discussion of the effect of this ruling and several others released this year indicates that it is raising questions about the public's confidence in the Supreme Court in particular and the judicial system as a whole.

While our experience with Covid provides a glimpse into the workings of the healthcare system, the controversy regarding the *Roe v. Wade* decision involves more significant revelations. It has caused people to question the long-standing assertion that Supreme Court judges are guided solely by the Constitution and established law. It served to unmask forces that shape the country's social institutions, including political ideology, religious beliefs, social and cultural values, and appreciation of the importance of scientific research. All of which worked to diminish the public's confidence. This has, in turn, furthered the steady decline in trust in the country's social institutions, which is noteworthy because, as we will see in the final chapter of the book, it has significant health implications.

Chapter 3

Private Health Insurance

The evolution of private health insurance in the United States is marked by two sudden growth spurts. The first occurred during the World War II era. The second came in response to the Patient Protection and Affordable Care Act (ACA), also known as Obamacare, which passed in 2010 and was implemented in 2014.

ORIGINS OF PRIVATE HEALTH INSURANCE

People didn't need health insurance when doctors accepted a fee for their services, and hospitals were places people were not ready to go to willingly. Surgeons did begin to admit some paying patients to hospitals during the first few decades of the twentieth century. Once the Great Depression hit in 1929, more people may have been willing to be hospitalized, but most couldn't afford it. Those admitted because of an emergency had difficulty paying for their stay.

An innovative solution surfaced when Baylor University Hospital in Dallas, Texas, realized that the category of patients most apt to default on payment were schoolteachers. The hospital came up with a plan to offset its losses. It offered the Dallas Board of Education a proposal whereby teachers could pay 50 cents per month for twenty-one days of hospital care per year if it was necessary. The plan was called Blue Cross.

The arrangement got a major boost during the war years due to the Stabilization Act of 1942, restricting employers' ability to raise wages. Employers responded by offering benefits to attract workers who were scarce because so many men had left to serve in the war. This occurrence marks the origins of employer-sponsored health insurance in this country. A ruling during the Eisenhower era locked employer-based insurance into place by making it tax-free for both the employer and the employee.

The Blue Shield plan came into existence not long after the Blue Cross plan. Originating in California, it was sponsored by doctors who thought hospitals were gaining too much say over healthcare delivery. Blue Cross and Blue Shield plans were sold separately until 1982, when they merged.

It didn't happen immediately, but after some experience with the Blue Cross reimbursement, critics began saying how it was structured aided and abetted hospitals in raising prices. Defenders said there were important benefits inherent in the arrangement. It allowed hospitals to increase the amount paid by those who were insured and use the extra funds to care for people who could not afford to be hospitalized. This was known as *cost shifting*. There was nothing underhanded or secret about it. It was the accustomed method doctors and hospitals used before rates for healthcare services became standardized.

In fact, the exorbitant amount hospitals charged a celebrity who had been hospitalized was likely to make headlines. The hospital was pleased to notify the press about it. The celebrity liked being known as someone willing to contribute to the care of those with less money. It made for good press for both.

Here's a lengthy aside with more information on how things worked—until costs got out of hand. Since Blue Cross would only pay for hospital care, doctors would routinely admit patients for tests. The catch was that, officially, Blue Cross would only pay for hospitalization if the patient was sick. Acknowledging this reality, doctors routinely admitted patients with a diagnosis that proved to be negative after the appropriate tests were performed. Consider the implications. It is less expensive to have tests done on people who walk in, have the test done, and go home. So, doctors ordered more tests to justify admitting the person to the hospital. Patients didn't object because they knew they wouldn't be charged for all the tests. Both doctors and patients could convince themselves that tests carried out in the hospital would be more accurate because patients could be monitored before and after getting tested. It was pretty obvious that there were a lot of healthy people being admitted. Hospitals had no reason to object to this practice because Blue Cross was in the business of reimbursing hospitals for whatever they charged. Eventually, healthcare costs did begin to climb, and people did start to complain about it. So, who's to blame for letting the situation get out of hand?

Another innovative health insurance arrangement came into existence in 1938 when Henry Kaiser took on the challenge of building the Los Angeles aqueduct. Workers were willing to do the dangerous work in an isolated setting only if they could be assured of having medical care readily available in case of accidents. No doctor would start a practice in such a setting without some assurances of his own, namely that he could make enough money to set up an office and meet living expenses. Kaiser's creative solution was to have his workers contribute 5 cents per day to guarantee the availability of medical care. He equipped a train car as a fully outfitted doctor's office to be moved along as work on the dam progressed. The doctor got the money paid by the workers regardless of whether they needed to see him or not.

This arrangement, known as *capitation*, proved so successful that Kaiser used it to attract workers during World War II to his shipyards and steel mills. He established a new organization, Kaiser Permanente, in 1942 to handle health insurance for his workers. When the war ended, Kaiser opened up the plan to the public. (You will see references to research conducted by the Kaiser Family Foundation throughout this discussion. The Kaiser Family Foundation has no connection to the Kaiser Permanente health insurance organization.)

While the American Medical Association (AMA) was not in favor of the Blue Cross–Blue Shield (BC-BS) plan, it was vehemently opposed to the Kaiser Permanente plan because doctors were essentially Kaiser plan employees. The AMA considered this completely unacceptable. It pressured hospitals to deny admitting privileges to doctors who accepted positions that involved capitation payment. That forced Kaiser Permanente to build its own hospitals. Over time, the Kaiser Permanente healthcare system dropped capitation and began employing doctors on a salaried basis.

It is worth noting that these health insurance organizations and others created during the first half of the twentieth century were nonprofit entities. There were no shareholders and no profits to distribute. If earnings exceeded projected costs, the "excess" was plowed back into the organization. That changed over the next few decades when healthcare costs started increasing at a greater rate than expected. The excess is now more likely to be invested in other profitable healthcare enterprises or held in an interest-bearing account.

FROM A COMMUNITY RATE TO RISK-RATING

Private, for-profit insurance companies, which sold life insurance, were fairly well established by the 1930s. They exhibited no interest in offering health insurance until World War II when the health insurance business took off. Consider how fast that business grew—in 1940, 9 percent of the population had hospital insurance; by 1950, the proportion had risen to 50 percent.[1] The new health insurance plans developed during this period were sponsored by well-established life insurance companies operating on a for-profit basis.

Both the BC-BS plans and the emergent for-profit health insurance companies could have tried to hold down costs, but there was not much pressure to do that. The post-war economy was booming, and healthcare costs were not rising very fast, which encouraged more private insurance companies to enter this market. As the field got more crowded, they began to compete by lowering premiums, basing them on "experience" or "risk-rating." In other words, they calculated how often particular categories of customers sought healthcare services and set the rate accordingly. Furthermore, they began aggressively recruiting customers less likely to run up high healthcare costs. This became known as "cherry-picking" and "cream-skimming."

It's perfectly obvious that you can attract more business by reducing the premium you charge, and the for-profit insurance companies were quick to figure out how to do that. They began marketing their plans to organizations employing younger, healthier workers with safe, quiet office jobs. There were no laws preventing companies from retiring their employees at the age of sixty-five, which was, in fact, the regular practice. Insurance companies were not concerned about signing up people who sat all day, probably smoked, and didn't get any exercise because the chances were good that they would not suffer ill health until after they retired (often shortly after they retired), and the company was no longer insuring them. Private health insurance companies had no trouble getting employers to adopt plans that cost less than BC-BS plans.

The nonprofit status of BC-BS plans prevented them from lowering their rates depending on the characteristics of buyers. They were set up to offer a community rate—the same rate to everyone enrolled in the plan.

Observers, seeing the success of the for-profit insurance companies, charged the Blues with being inefficient and advised them to adopt business practices. The Blues moved slowly to embrace the message, but they picked up the pace over time. They began consolidating their operations through mergers, acquisitions, and joint ventures with various for-profit organizations.

The history of the Anthem health insurance company serves as a good example. It was one of the first companies to begin expanding its operations. It started by developing a relationship with the Blues in Indiana in the late 1940s. Over the next few decades, it absorbed the New Hampshire, Colorado, Nevada, and Maine Blues. It operated as a mutual insurance company, meaning it was owned by policyholders, and profits were supposed to be returned to policyholders in the form of lower premiums. It turned itself into a for-profit entity in 2001. In 2004, it merged with Wellpoint, which represented the California Blues. Both organizations had been acquiring other kinds of healthcare enterprises along the way. Anthem changed its name to Elevance in 2022.

It is worth noting that, according to Forbes, as of 2022, Kaiser Permanente was the largest health insurer in the country with 8.2 million enrollees, and Elevance was the second largest with 4.7 million enrollees.[2]

The fact that healthcare organizations were rapidly becoming more business-like was in line with the increasing pressure on the part of some to argue that the provision of healthcare services worked best in response to market forces, that is, supply and demand. Patients were to be considered *consumers*, who were expected to shop for medical goods and services just as they shopped for other products. This was in line with the "consumer-driven healthcare" movement that started in the 1970s and was in high gear by the 1990s. The label may not be as popular these days as it was then, but the basic ideas behind it continue to be promoted.

FROM PREPAID CARE TO HEALTH MAINTENANCE

The prepaid care health insurance model, pioneered by the Blues and Kaiser, got an enormous boost from legislation passed in 1974. This occurred because President Nixon was searching for a way to put limits on the growth of medical care costs. Advocates argued that prepaid care would result in savings because the arrangement would permit patients to seek care earlier before their problems became more complicated and more costly to treat. So, not only would such an approach save money, but it would also have health benefits. President Nixon presented the plan to the country as something that would help people *maintain* their health, which is where the *health maintenance* label comes from. That did not stop the medical establishment from objecting to the prepayment feature of this legislation. The AMA labeled it "socialized medicine" in a massive media campaign. The AMA's objections notwithstanding, legislation requiring employers to offer this option to their employees and funding to support start-up costs passed. This is also when the term "health maintenance organization," or HMO, came into widespread use.

The way HMOs were designed to work was that both patients and doctors would sign up with a particular HMO. Doctors would do so by signing a contract. The earliest HMOs paid doctors a salary; others offered doctors a contract specifying a fixed amount of money per capita—a capitation fee. There was no restriction on doctors signing up with more than one HMO. Patients would sign on by "enrolling" in a single plan that employers had agreed to offer as an option. The employer would contract with the HMO agreeing to pay a fixed amount of money, the *premium*, to which the employee would contribute an amount determined by the employer.

The fact that the legislation made a considerable amount of money available for start-up costs brought many new parties into the health maintenance business. Initially, the new HMOs used Kaiser Permanente as their model for establishing themselves as nonprofit organizations. It did not take long for that to change. Some HMOs were created with the understanding that producing a profit for their owners was precisely what the owners had in mind.

Many new HMOs, both for-profit and nonprofit, were established without enough planning, funding, or thought given to administration. Some of the struggling HMOs were bought out. Others simply closed up shop and disappeared. In either case, patients had to sign up with another, possibly new and untested organization, with new doctors, different rules, and so on. This was when the idea that the healthcare sector was inefficient, lacking in managerial talent, and backward in the application of the latest business techniques really took hold. It was also when all those health sector organizations became more aggressive in their efforts to operate more efficiently to gain a greater market share, that is, more prospective patients.

It is worth noting that the Kaiser Permanente plan was established with the aim of providing both continuing and preventive care by relying more heavily on care provided by generalists or primary care practitioners (PCPs) as opposed to specialists or surgeons. It could do this because it hired the physicians who worked there. The newly established HMOs adopted this strategy as well. Internists, pediatricians, and family practitioners, the PCPs, were to act as gatekeepers. They were expected to treat most of the patient's problems—referring patients to a specialist only if a problem truly required considerably more specialized knowledge. By monitoring the patient's care more closely, gatekeepers were to keep patients out of the hospital, which is beneficial to the patient (unless, of course, that effort becomes too restrictive).

Primary care doctors reacted by complaining that the HMOs were imposing too many restrictions on what they could do, pressuring them to see more patients than they could handle, imposing time limits on patient visits, and so on.

It took a few more years for executives of the newly established HMOs to realize that one of the main obstacles they faced in trying to control costs or, more importantly, make a profit was that the HMO could only control the costs of care taking place within the doctor's office. However, the HMO lost control once patients were admitted to the hospital. HMOs had contracts with hospitals covering basic costs per day but could not control the additional costs incurred once the patient was admitted. Thus, things like how long a patient was there, what tests were performed, and how many times tests were repeated, which all have a significant impact on costs, were not under the control of the HMO. The move to manage the patient's care at all stages of treatment brings us to the next iteration in the process—the era of *managed care*.

The concepts economists use to explain the operations of private sector organizations apply here. As HMOs became larger and more powerful, they were able to demand better deals in negotiations with hospitals and all the companies from which they order equipment and supplies (economies of scale). In many cases, managed care organizations could and ultimately did simply buy out their suppliers (vertical integration). This created even larger and more powerful organizations. Business executives argued that it was self-evident that "competition is healthy!" And that explains how the labels shifted from *managed care* and *health maintenance* to *managed competition*. Managed competition was the foundational idea on which the Clinton health-care reform plan was based. The managed competition concept was tainted by the failure of the Clinton healthcare reform proposal and fell into disfavor. Health insurance companies announced that they would prefer their offerings to be known as "healthcare plans."

Curiously, even though employers had seen little evidence that managed care was reducing costs during the 1980s, they suddenly became convinced that managed care was the way to go during the 1990s. Employers began dropping traditional fee-for-service insurance plans and offering only health maintenance benefit packages. In 1993, roughly half of American workers (versus the population as a whole) were enrolled in managed care programs; by 1995, that figure leaped to 73 percent.[3] The speed of the shift surprised everyone. While arguments about the pros and cons of managed care did not cease, the number of people enrolled in health maintenance plans increased steadily through the decade of the 1990s.

But this is when enrollees began expressing a rising level of dissatisfaction with the HMO model. While they were unhappy about the increasing costs, they were registering most displeasure about the rules imposed by HMOs, especially restrictions on which doctors they could see and how long they could stay in the hospital. The charge against HMOs popularized during this period was that patients were being discharged "quicker and sicker." By 1996, twenty-nine states had passed laws governing early discharge. The rising level of dissatisfaction led managed care organizations to introduce a variation known as the "preferred provider organization," or PPO. The PPO option allowed enrollees to pay a higher premium for the right to select doctors of their own choosing. When that adjustment did not fully overcome enrollee dissatisfaction, a "point-of-service" (POS) option appeared. This required the enrollee to select a primary care physician from the approved list, now known as a *network*, who would assume responsibility for recommending a specialist, if necessary. The POS was offered at a higher premium than the HMO premium, but it was one that was lower than the PPO option.

The next iteration was the EPO, which stands for Exclusive Provider Organization. It is like an HMO in that care outside the network is not covered. However, EPOs generally permit enrollees to refer themselves to a specialist within the network.

Critics were ready to point out that the alternative arrangements gave employers an excuse to revise benefit plans and pass on a larger proportion of the premium to employees. Health plan companies took the opportunity to promote the PPO, POS, and EPO as innovations rising out of the preferences consumers were registering, presenting it all as the new era of "consumer-driven health care." This is a concept that keeps coming up even when not labeled exactly that way.

By the end of the 1990s, health insurance companies conceived of a new option claiming it was in response to consumer demand for plans with lower premiums. This turned out to be a *high-deductible plan*. The companies convinced Congress to pass legislation in 2003 linking high-deductible plans to health savings accounts (HSAs). The idea was that the HSAs would allow enrollees to set aside a certain amount of income in tax-free accounts that could be used to cover medical costs. Such plans would have lower premiums because insurance coverage would start after the enrollee spent a substantial amount of money out-of-pocket—the *deductible*. Depending on the plan, this could be $1,000, $2,000, $5,000, or more.

The 2023 HSA tax-free contribution, which can roll over from year to year, is $3,850 for an individual and $7,750 for a family. There is a cap on total out-of-pocket expenditures (this includes the deductible, copayments, and coinsurance). As of 2023, the cap is $9,100 for an individual and $18,200 for a family. Critics reacted by saying that the high-deductible plan, together with the HSA, amounts to another tax loophole, advantageous to the rich and not something that benefits the majority of Americans.

THE AFFORDABLE CARE ACT

The Affordable Care Act (ACA), also known as Obamacare, of 2010 is the most significant healthcare coverage development since Medicare and Medicaid legislation was enacted in 1965. (More on that in the next chapter.) It also marks the second turning point or phase in the development of private health insurance.

Although the ACA is now well-accepted, it was unpopular with a large segment of the population when it came into existence and for quite a few years after that. People said they liked their health arrangements and didn't want anything changed by the new law. Conservative members of Congress did their best to discredit the plan. When they found that labeling it as "socialism" was not enough, they ran ads claiming it would create "death panels" with the power to decide whether elderly patients received health care or were left to die. Republicans introduced bills in Congress aimed at overturning the ACA over fifty times between 2010 and 2016. They lost every time.

By contrast, major stakeholders, including groups representing physicians, hospitals, and insurance companies, were not opposed to the legislation as long as it was not a total government takeover. They said that the country's healthcare arrangements needed to be more orderly, and it was time for that to happen.

How the framers of the ACA legislation succeeded in creating a plan that introduced significant changes in the country's healthcare system in the face of considerable opposition deserves closer attention. What they achieved is a testament to political shrewdness.

The authors of the legislation started with the understanding that they had four options from which to choose, as outlined by the Institute of Medicine (IOM). As you will recall from the previous chapter, the IOM is nonpolitical. It relies on experts to address specific problems it is charged with addressing.

The four options outlined by the IOM were as follows:

1. An *employer mandate* requires employers to provide insurance for all employees and all others to be covered by public plans;
2. An *individual mandate* requires everyone to buy their own insurance with the aid of tax credits;
3. An *incremental approach*, that is, expansion of existing public programs—Medicare, Medicaid, and Children's Health Insurance Program (CHIP)—plus government assistance to allow the uninsured to buy into these programs; and
4. The *single-payer plan*.

What makes the ACA so extraordinary is that it succeeded in rolling the first three alternatives into one proposal, leaving out only the fourth option, the single-payer plan. There was also some discussion of a public plan operated under federal government auspices established to compete with for-profit plans. The public plan idea did not move forward. However, it has not disappeared and continues to be discussed by health policy types. Similarly, it is worth noting that while the single-payer option produced the most vigorous opposition at the time and continues to do so, that isn't stopping proponents from proposing bills to have it implemented on a regular basis.

What the framers of the ACA legislation succeeded in doing is bundling a liberal goal—health insurance coverage for everyone—together with a conservative approach to insurance, that is, personal responsibility for selecting a private health plan of one's own choosing. That allowed the *individual mandate*, requiring everyone to buy health insurance, to go forward. The *employer mandate*, which would have the most impact on small employers, could be included because the government would provide tax relief for small employers to ease the financial burden. The law expanded government programs but left control over the provision of health insurance mainly in the hands of the private sector.

What is interesting to reflect on is that public opinion surveys indicate that some elements in the plan were popular from the beginning across political lines, even if the plan itself remained unpopular. This includes coverage for pre-existing conditions, preventive care, financial help to assist moderate and low-income families in purchasing insurance, and coverage for young adults to age twenty-six on their parents' plans.

Let's look at the individual mandate first, the least popular part of the ACA, or the most objectionable part, if you prefer.

THE INDIVIDUAL MANDATE

Before 2010, insurance companies were under no obligation to sell insurance to everyone who applied for it. From the perspective of insurance companies, enrolling individuals is much riskier than enrolling a large number of employees working for a company. What if the individual turned out to have an undiagnosed pre-existing health problem that would require continuous testing and treatment? Why accept such a risk if you don't have to?

That meant individuals had a difficult time getting insurance. Why they were interested in seeking insurance in the first place was clear: They lacked bargaining power. That is still the case. Most of us would go to the emergency room or agree to life-saving surgery during the crisis even if we had no insurance without weighing the costs and benefits, right? We would not be considering the fact that the bill would very likely be a lot higher than it would be for someone with health insurance. Uninsured persons were and are still billed at the full rate, which amounts to whatever the hospital wants to charge. That amount is nothing like the rate the hospital and insurance company agree to through a negotiated contract. The uninsured patient may be able to get a reduction in charges after the fact, but there is no assurance the hospital will agree.

The ACA imposed fines on individuals to stop them from opting out of obtaining health insurance. The penalty amount was to be phased in once the law was implemented at $95 per person in 2014 or 1 percent of taxable income up to 2.5 percent of taxable income up to a maximum of $2,085 per family.

The rationale for requiring all individuals to purchase health insurance was to prevent people from buying insurance only when they found they needed it. As some pundits put it, this would be like deciding to buy while in the ambulance on the way to the hospital. Allowing people to avoid paying until they need health care is obviously not fair to all those who have paid their share all along. Furthermore, having healthy people as well as sick people in the insurance pool spreads the risk—to the insurer. This was a cornerstone on which both the BC-BS and the Kaiser Permanente plans were founded. And it is the basis on which private insurance operates when it lowers costs to companies that employ persons who are estimated to pose a lower risk.

However, Congress repealed the penalty in 2019. It is in force in four states and Washington, DC. The amount of the fine varies.

Another significant requirement imposed by the ACA was that states set up Health Insurance Marketplaces where individuals not eligible for either government-sponsored or employer-sponsored insurance could shop for health insurance remains intact. The federal government distributed $4 billion in start-up funds for this purpose.

The ACA standardized the policies that were to be sold through state health marketplaces. This was meant to increase transparency in how the plans worked. Insurance companies, licensed by the state, can sell one or more of the policies and charge whatever they want but are not permitted to alter the structure of plans. The basic difference in the four levels is the balance in the contribution the insurance company makes versus what the enrollee pays for medical care services.

Bronze plan—insurance company covers 60 percent, and enrollee pays 40 percent

Silver plan—insurance company covers 70 percent, and enrollee pays 30 percent

Gold plan—insurance company covers 80 percent, and enrollee pays 20 percent

Platinum plan—insurance company covers 90 percent, and enrollee pays 10 percent

A catastrophic plan is available to individuals under the age of thirty and others under special conditions. It is inexpensive but covers only three primary care visits.

The higher the value of the metal, the higher the monthly premium, but the lower the copayments. The deductible, which varies depending on the characteristics of enrollees, is set by the insurance carrier. It is higher for lower-metal-value plans. The government sets a cap on the total out-of-pocket expenditures for which enrollees in all plans are responsible. While the cap may be lower for some plans, as of 2023, it may not exceed $1,800 for individuals and $18,700 for families.

The law made cost-sharing arrangements available to qualified individuals who signed up for the Silver plan. Enrollees with incomes between 100 and 400 percent of poverty qualify for *tax credits* to reduce the monthly premium cost or as a tax rebate at the end of the tax year. The law made insurance *tax subsidies* available to persons whose earnings are under 250 percent of poverty. Those whose incomes fall under 138 percent of poverty can sign up for Medicaid coverage through the health marketplace in states that extended Medicaid.

There are quite a few other rules applying to insurers, such as the prohibition against using pre-existing health conditions in setting rates, imposing lifetime limits on coverage, and rescinding coverage except in cases of fraud.

Because the Supreme Court found the Medicaid expansion section of the ACA to be unconstitutional, states could keep the Medicaid funds they were already receiving without expanding their Medicaid programs or setting up the state insurance marketplaces. (More about Medicaid in chapter 4.) While some states refused to cooperate, others said they were willing but not equipped to create a state marketplace. The federal government proceeded to set up health insurance marketplaces for states that couldn't or wouldn't do it on their own. The result was that twenty-seven states ended up with federally supported marketplaces; ten entered into partnerships with the federal government; and fourteen set up state-based marketplaces. (That's fifty states plus Washington, DC.)

It did not take long for the federal government to discover that people were confused about how the marketplaces worked. They were not sure whether they were entitled to tax credits or tax subsidies, not sure where to get information and help to understand what the plans they were signing up for covered, and not sure how to go about it all. The fact that insurance companies offered multiple plans under each metal made things even more confusing. The number of plans ran into the hundreds. The solution the government came up with was to provide states with funds to train people to serve as helpers called *navigators*—to help people "navigate" the health insurance marketplace. (The Trump administration cut funding for navigators. The Biden administration reinstated it.)

As an aside, returning to the notion that "consumer-driven" health care would shape healthcare arrangements, health marketplaces quickly made clear that shopping for health insurance products was not something consumers were prepared to do on their own.

THE EMPLOYER MANDATE

Most people in this country have health insurance coverage through their employers, which has been true since it was introduced during the World War II era. The government started collecting statistics on the number of people who had private health insurance in 1959 but didn't do so on an annual basis until 1989. Private health insurance peaked around 1984 when 76.8 percent of the population had some form of private health insurance. According to the US Census Bureau, that dropped to 66 percent as of 2021, with 54.3 percent of those with private insurance covered by employer-based insurance.

When the details of the ACA requirements first came out, many people were surprised to discover that employers had been under no obligation to offer health insurance to their employees before then. The vast majority of large employers did so voluntarily. With the passage of the ACA, employers with 200 employees or more were required to provide health insurance by law. Not doing so carried a $2,000 penalty per employee after the first thirty employees. As of 2022, the penalty is $2,750 per employee.

Some employers said they would accept the penalty because it was less expensive than paying for health insurance. It seems that few carried through with that threat. (There are no data on this. But one can imagine that they might have had second thoughts when they considered that they would have difficulty recruiting workers. Who would work for such a company if other companies provided the benefit?)

Small companies were especially opposed to the ACA requirement that they provide health insurance to their employees because insurance companies charged them much more based on the unpredictability of risk. Small companies said they couldn't afford it. The ACA addressed the problem by creating the Small Business Health Options Plan (SHOP). Employers with fewer than fifty employees could apply to the SHOP plan for assistance in finding a plan. Employers with twenty-five or fewer employees whose average wages fell under $53,000 could get up to a 50 percent tax credit through SHOP. (Eighteen SHOP plans are operated by states and have slightly different rules than the plan operated by the federal government.)

The ACA legislation specified that employers were expected to provide health insurance coverage for full-time employees. That led some employers to cut employee work hours to under thirty hours per week, turning those employees into part-time workers no longer needing to be covered. Other major employers, such as those in Silicon Valley, used another approach. They opted to employ some people on a contractual basis, meaning those workers are not employees and receive no company benefits. Contract workers are required to obtain health insurance on their own.

As of 1986, those who either lost their jobs or quit could turn to COBRA (the Consolidated Omnibus Budget Reconciliation Act), which requires insurance companies to provide continued coverage for eighteen months after the employee leaves their place of employment. The legislation did not address costs, meaning that insurance companies could charge the full cost for continued coverage.

Critics have been objecting to employer-sponsored health insurance for almost as long as it's been in existence. The primary criticism was that it was responsible for "job lock." The idea was that people felt trapped in jobs they didn't want to be in but had to stay with because they would lose their health insurance if they quit. The existence of state health insurance marketplaces ended job lock a decade ago. However, it seems that escaping job lock was not something people were ready to take advantage of until the workplace shutdown caused by the Covid epidemic. The Covid experience had the effect of causing workers to act on the realization of what they didn't like about their jobs and that it was a good time to quit. One of the reasons (I'm not suggesting it is the main reason, but still . . .) that so many employees quit during the Covid lockdown was that the state health insurance marketplace made it possible to obtain health insurance outside of the workplace.

Some would argue that the demise of employer-sponsored health insurance may be closer than policymakers would have predicted before the onset of Covid. In an article in the *Harvard Business Review*, one observer claims that the new generation of tech-savvy workers, who are ready to change jobs far more often than their predecessors, won't be putting up with the cost and inconvenience associated with employer-sponsored insurance much longer. He points out that "When they switch jobs mid-year, they've already met their health insurance deductible on their previous employer's plan, they must effectively start over under their new employer's plan."[4]

Another consideration is the recognition that employer-sponsored health insurance is not the great deal it was in the past. Ten years ago, the average single premium was $5,615; the average family premium was $15,745. "The average premium for family coverage increased 20% over the next five years and 43% over the last ten years."[5] The average annual premium for single coverage in 2022 was $7,911 and $22,463 for family coverage. Employers have been raising the proportion of the premium they expect employees to pay. And there are still additional costs beyond the premium, starting with the deductible, plus a copay for doctors' visits and prescription drugs. The average deductible in 2022 for single coverage was $1,763, meaning it increased by 17 percent over the last five years and 61 percent over the previous ten years. Wages have not kept up with these increases.

We'll just have to see when and if the employer-sponsored health insurance arrangement will change. Some critics argue that the tax benefit employers enjoy is keeping the arrangement in place even though it is a huge administrative burden.

As an aside, what do you think? Is the fact that employers do not pay taxes on the money they set aside to pay for health insurance enough of an incentive to prevent its demise? Or is it something else? Without employer-sponsored health insurance, all those private insurance corporations would lose a lot of business. And the country might choose to move into something closer to a vast public health insurance plan, like *Medicare-for-all*, which some claim is *socialism* and find totally objectionable. Are employers and/or employees holding on to the employer-sponsored arrangement to prevent that? Or is that conspiratorial thinking and the absence of change in employer-based health insurance arrangements come closer to being a matter of inertia?

HEALTH INSURANCE AND PRICES

Rising healthcare prices, in general, and health insurance costs, in particular, constitute continuing public concerns. The question is not only what can be done about the high costs but who should do it. We've already tried piling the responsibility on consumers and found that that didn't work nearly as well as proponents said it would. Researchers report that consumers simply aren't willing to shop for less costly health insurance plans from year to year.[6]

Turning to what the private sector can do to control healthcare costs, let's focus first on employers and second on the health insurance industry. In 2018, some very big names in the private sector—Warren Buffet, Jeff Bezos, and Jamie Dimon—attempted to mount a challenge to the dominance of health insurance companies by creating an insurance company of their own, Haven, which they said would operate "free from profit incentives and constraints." Haven lasted three years. According to some commentators, these corporate titans found that "It's the Prices, Stupid." This was a slogan popularized by some highly regarded economists in 2003, referring to what doctors and hospitals charge for healthcare goods and services. And it is the prices that, as it turns out, Haven didn't have the power to alter. Health insurance industry representatives have been saying for some time that they have tried negotiating over prices with major hospital networks but that those networks have gotten so big and so powerful that even the biggest health insurers have been unable to do anything about rising prices.

As an aside, the author of the slogan, "It's the Prices, Stupid," Uwe Reinhardt, who was for many years recognized as the leading health economist in the country, has had more to say about this country's healthcare arrangements.[7] He pointed out that one of the main obstacles standing in the way of creating a successful healthcare system in this country is the absence of discussion on ethics. In his view, we must first decide whether health care is a right. He states that our inability to come to that conclusion results in not only high ethical costs but high economic costs as well.

Quite a few large employers have taken steps to reduce their costs by establishing self-funded arrangements and hiring insurance companies to process claims. Under this arrangement, the large company assumes the financial risk of providing healthcare benefits for its employees. To insure against unexpected costs, the companies buy "stop-loss" insurance to cover reimbursement above a specified dollar amount. Such contracts are governed by the Employee Retirement Income Security Act (ERISA), established to protect retirement funds from mismanagement. It limits government oversight to the federal level. This avoids taxation by the state. It is also true any savings achieved under this arrangement hasn't resulted in a reduction in the price employees pay for their insurance.

What about health insurance companies—is there anything they can do to lower consumer costs? Some have taken steps to lower their costs, which has not been particularly advantageous to the enrollees. For example, hospitals and healthcare systems may achieve higher earnings by *overtreating*—that is, providing more care than the patient needs.[8] Some insurance companies are doing just the opposite, embracing an *undertreating* approach and denying claims. One study of marketplace insurers found that they denied nearly one in five claims in 2020. The denial rates varied across insurers "from a low of 1% to a high of 80%."[9] The researchers who reported these findings say that relatively few denials include a specific reason, with 72 percent falling into the category of "all other reasons." They found that few consumers appealed such decisions. The fact that denials vary so much suggests there is no fixed standard for denials, an issue that seems worth looking into.

Before getting deeper into what insurance companies can or should do to control costs, it is important to reflect on the fact that health insurance companies are profit-making enterprises. And the primary objective of all for-profit organizations is making money. It is their "legal, ethical, and fiduciary responsibility" to do so.[10] It is worth recalling how this works. When Medicare was passed, health insurance companies were permitted to charge 8.4 percent over the cost of traditional Medicare, but health insurance companies were routinely setting aside considerably more than that. The ACA fixed the amount companies could claim for administration and profit, known as the *medical-loss ratio*, at 15 percent for large group plans and 20 percent in the individual and small group market. Health insurance companies refer to the money spent on medical care as the *loss* part of the medical-*loss* ratio. The money spent on medical care carries a negative label because of its negative impact on the bottom line. The logic inherent in that concept is obvious— increase profits by cutting *medical care* costs.

This ACA ruling means that companies earning more are expected to return anything over that percentage to enrollees in the form of a rebate. That is exactly what was supposed to happen as a result of windfall profits insurance companies made while Covid was raging and patients weren't going to hospitals for elective procedures. The estimate was that $2.7 billion would be returned in rebates in 2022. The extent to which that happened is difficult to monitor.

What did become clear is that the health insurance industry's profits during the Covid epidemic were impressive. To wit, UnitedHealth Group led the field in profitability in the first half of 2022, bringing in $10.1 billion in profit. But health insurance companies were also reporting huge profits before the onset of Covid. The question of what accounts for the profitability of the health insurance industry is a topic that is regularly debated. The answer depends on who you ask. Spokespersons for the industry state that it is due to practices designed to achieve increased efficiency. Critics argue that the primary mechanism the industry has employed depends less on efficiency than consolidation with the aim of increasing market share. There is good reason to argue that the five largest health insurance companies got to where they are because of numerous previous mergers. "UnitedHealth Group and CVS Health are by far the most vertically integrated companies among the major national payers, with each encompassing a sprawling enterprise with a slew of diverse businesses under its umbrella."[11]

When the wave of mergers first began to gain momentum a few decades ago, the Federal Trade Commission (FTC) and quite a few states' attorneys took notice. The FTC's concern was that certain mergers would produce organizations so large that their size would result in restraint of trade, that they would be the major and perhaps only insurer in the area. States' attorneys were afraid enrollees in their states would have little choice in selecting an insurance plan and that there would be no competition to keep insurance costs in check. The upshot was the creation of the US Department of Justice and Federal Trade Commission Horizontal Merger Guidelines in 1997. Critics say that the government has done little to prevent mergers since then, so a single insurer now monopolizes too many markets.[12]

Another criticism of health insurance company operations that surfaces with some regularity has to do with the compensation awarded to company executives. Although the story behind the 2003 package that went to Aetna's CEO, John Rowe, may be dated, I find it to be particularly engaging.[13]

While Rowe's compensation package was not atypical, his case had a special twist. He received $1,042,146 in salary, a $2.2 million bonus, new stock options estimated to be worth $5.6 million, and a $7 million cash payment on stock options, plus other compensation of nearly $400,000—a staggering $16,242,146 in total. Other officers of the company received huge compensation packages as well that year. One group of investors decided to take action. The United Association of Plumbers, Pipefitters & Sprinkler Fitters proposed that Aetna's board of directors and shareholders limit Rowe's compensation package to $1 million and his annual bonuses be linked to performance measures. The board rejected the proposal, saying that it was too rigid. The union's move was spurred on by the company's decision to fire 10,700 employees and lay off an additional 700 over the previous year.

Compensation going to health insurance company CEOs is a regular feature in business publications. The highest paid CEOs in 2021 working for the following health insurance companies were paid as follows: Centene, $20.6

million; Molina Healthcare, $20 million; Cigna, $19.9 million; Elevance, $19.3 million; UnitedHealth Group, $18.4 million; and Humana, $16.5 million. While those are eye-popping numbers, it is also true, as some commentators point out, that CEOs in other industries earn even more. Salaries are merely competitive, they say.

Both health insurance CEO salaries and company profits provide fodder for continuing debate. While some observers are appalled by health insurance company profits, others point out that they actually make a modest profit, consistently falling in the 3 to 4 percent range, as compared to companies in some other sectors, such as banking which was estimated to have achieved a 30 percent profit in 2022. More recently, the profits made by gas and petroleum companies over the previous year—the year of high gas prices—have been in the headlines.

Assertions that other industries achieve greater profits are dismissed by critics who ask whether it is defensible for healthcare insurance companies and/or other healthcare organizations to be in the business of making a profit. To put it more starkly, some have asked—how much profit is reasonable when dealing with people's pain and suffering?

LEGISLATION AIMED AT HEALTH SYSTEM REFORM

The ACA failed to achieve its primary objective, universal health insurance coverage. Based on 2021 figures, it did, however, reduce the number of uninsured Americans by 31 million. The uninsured rate now stands at an all-time low of 8 percent. The number of people enrolled in individual market plans reached 19.8 million in 2015 but dropped to 14.1 million by 2020. Passage of the American Rescue Plan Act (ARPA) of 2021, together with enhanced subsidies, boosted outreach, and an extended enrollment period, brought enrollment up to 16.9 million by 2022.[14] The ARPA was designed to be in effect through 2022 and has not been renewed. The expected increase in the uninsurance rate is something that is certain to receive more attention over the following year.

Two other issues continue to attract the attention of health policy analysts—underinsurance and medical debt. There is general agreement on how underinsurance is defined: persons who spend more than 10 percent of their income, 5 percent if they are low income, on health care, excluding premiums. Or if their deductible is greater than 5 percent of their income. How many people fall into this category is not easy to establish since how medical debt accrues varies tremendously. Some people end up with credit card debt, some mortgage their homes, and some take out loans. About a quarter of working-age adults were estimated to be underinsured prior to legislation extending health insurance coverage passed in response to the Covid epidemic. A national study conducted in 2022 revealed that about four in ten Americans have medical debt.[15] Making the problem worse, in some cases, accounts are sent to collections agencies, which has harmful consequences that can be hard to overcome, including difficulty getting a job. Medical debt is the single most common cause of bankruptcy.

Underinsurance is closely connected to medical debt and affects more Americans than one might guess. Those who are underinsured consume less health care. That does not turn out to be a savings to them or the country's healthcare budget because their health problems usually don't go away on their own and instead show up as more serious and more costly to treat later.

So, after everything you've learned about how private health insurance works, I leave you to decide how efficient and effective it is in delivering what it promises. What about the effect of competition across multiple health insurance plans? Plans with different rules that apply to so many different categories of people? How beneficial is that to prospective enrollees? If the preceding discussion seems to provide no clear answers, you are not alone in coming to that conclusion. Be assured that how the private health insurance system operates in this country is a source of never-ending discourse among health policy analysts. The debate is further fueled by evidence of the growing role of private equity investment in the healthcare sector, which you will hear more about in the chapters to follow.[16] These are folks whose primary objective is to invest in a sector that is sure to produce a profit.

Chapter 4

Health Insurance— Public Programs

The US Census Bureau report on health insurance coverage indicates that, as of 2021, the majority of people in this country, at 66 percent, were covered by private health insurance policies, 35.7 percent had government-sponsored insurance, and 8.3 percent were uninsured. Of those with government-sponsored health insurance, 18.9 percent were covered by Medicaid, and Medicare covered 18.4 percent. The rest were covered by other government-sponsored health insurance plans, including those offered by the Veterans Administration (VA), Federal Employees (FEHB), military (TRICARE), and the Indian Health Service (IHS).

ORIGINS OF MEDICARE AND MEDICAID

When Medicare and Medicaid were first being considered, the post–World War II economy was booming, and the public was ready and willing to see social welfare programs created to overcome poverty. However, the government didn't have a measure for counting the number of people requiring social assistance. It had to determine who qualified and how many people this involved. The solution came about in 1963 when Mollie Orshansky of the Social Services Administration developed the poverty thresholds indicator. (You are sure to be amazed to hear what was considered a necessity and the assumptions she used in her calculations—for example, that men required a higher level of financial support than women because men were incapable of preparing their own meals. I recommend reading the short historical account presented by the US Census Bureau to see what goods and services are included because, amazingly, it is, with a few changes, the formula we use today.) Debates about the accuracy of the measure erupted immediately and have never stopped.

The government has announced the poverty line based on that formula every year since then. As of 2023, it stood at $13,590 for individuals and $27,750 for a family of four.

When government statisticians carried out a count of poor people for the first time, they were surprised to find an unexpectedly high number of Americans with incomes below the newly established, now-official poverty line. Various social welfare proposals designed to address the problem were introduced. Quite a few were implemented.

Policymakers knew that poor Americans were having difficulty paying for healthcare services. Not only were they unable to afford to buy their own health insurance, but it was not readily available to them then. The government proposed to institute two health insurance programs targeted at selected categories of poor people. Medicare was designed to provide health insurance for elderly members of society, that is, people over age sixty-five, who the government found to be the poorest category at that time. Medicaid was for poor women with small children. The State Children's Health Insurance Program (SCHIP), renamed CHIP, was established in 1997. It was to provide health insurance coverage for poor children under the age of nineteen in recognition of the fact that, by then, those over sixty-five were no longer the poorest members of society. Children were.

MEDICARE

The Medicare program was legislated as an amendment (Title 18) to the Social Security Act in 1965 with a budget of about $10 billion. As of 2020–2021, the budget stood at $829.5 billion and enrolled 63.9 million people.

Medicare was initially established as a two-part program: Part A was the hospital insurance portion, and Part B was to cover physicians' fees. Two additional parts, Parts C and D, were added later. Part C, now known as Medicare-Advantage, allows people to join Medicare-approved plans offered by private insurance companies that combine Parts A and B and typically include Part D. Part D, the prescription drug plan, was legislated in 2003. Part D plans are sold by private companies.

An open enrollment period that currently runs from October 15 to December 7 allows anyone who wishes to enroll in or change Medicare plans to do so. Penalties may apply for not signing up when a person first becomes eligible.

Anyone who has paid into the social security fund or Railroad Retirement Board for ten years or more is automatically eligible for Part A. People must sign up for Part B. The government outlines all the Medicare plan components in a manual that is updated annually. A hard copy is sent to all enrollees.

The information is also made available on the Medicare website as well as a variety of other websites. The amount of detail is overwhelming. What follows is an overview of the plan for 2023. It does not take into account all the special conditions, exceptions, and variations which go on and on.

Part A

Part A is funded through the 1.45 percent employee payroll deduction plus a 1.45 percent contribution on the employer's part over the person's work history. Part A covers hospitalization, skilled nursing home care, hospice care, and home health care. The Medicare site refers people interested in hospice and home health care to other websites.

There is a $1,600 deductible for each hospital stay. Nursing home coverage is free for the first twenty days after three days or more of hospitalization. For days twenty-one through one hundred, the person must pay $200 per day if Medicare approves the stay. There is a lifetime reserve of sixty days after day ninety. After the lifetime reserve days are used up, the person pays all costs.

Medicare Part A funding is held in reserve by the Medicare Trust Fund. The fiscal state of the Fund was getting considerable attention but was overshadowed by other sociopolitical concerns over the last few years. Medicare trustees report that expenditures are expected to exceed revenue by 2023. Assuming this continues, the Medicare Trust Fund will be depleted by 2028. Needless to say, this requires serious attention.

Part B

People do not receive Part B benefits automatically. A person must qualify for Social Security benefits first, a process that comes with its own rules, rules that are not complicated but must be followed. Signing up for Medicare Part B means the person agrees to pay an annual deductible of $226 plus a monthly premium taken from the enrollee's monthly social security check (not payroll check). Medicare states that most people pay the standard premium of $165 per month, which applies to individuals whose annual income is under $97,000. But there are six gradations that apply to higher earners, increasing to $561 per month for those earning over $500,000 per year. Finally, enrollees are charged a $10 copayment for each healthcare service visit.

Medicare lists all the healthcare services it covers in its publications. It also lists what it does not cover: dental care, eye exams for glasses, hearing aids, and cosmetic surgery, to name a few notable items.

Supplementary health insurance called Medigap came into existence because coinsurance and deductibles can run into a lot of money. There are ten standardized Medigap plans approved by the government (the number has varied from year to year as some were discontinued). They can be sold by any private insurance company that wishes to offer one or more of them. The sellers can charge what they wish. However, they cannot claim that they will provide something other than what is specified by the plan under that letter. This was done to eliminate what we think of as the "fine print."

Let's turn to Part D, the drug plan, next. (We will focus on Part C later in a separate section because it has received a great deal of attention of late and is generating considerable controversy.)

Part D

Medicare Part D was authorized by the Medicare Prescription Drug, Improvement, and Modernization Act, signed into law in 2003 at a cost of $395 billion. Two months later, the George W. Bush White House announced that it had recalculated that figure and found that it would actually cost $534 billion.[1] That caused some concern, but the legislation went into effect in 2006 as planned. Unfortunately, the proposed legislation came at a time when the costs of the war in Iraq were running higher than predicted, and the economy was not improving as fast as the White House said it would.

Part D plans are sold by insurance companies on a state-by-state basis. When the legislation first went into effect in 2007, there were 1,866 plans to choose from. The number dropped the following year and continued to drop over the next decade. The number of plans stands at 766 as of 2022, with an average of thirty-nine plans available in each state.

A unique feature of the original plan, the *donut hole*, was the result of a compromise reached by Congress because there was not enough money for full coverage. During its first year of operation, it worked as follows: The plan covered 75 percent of drug costs up to $2,250. After that, the person was expected to pay 100 percent for drugs—while in the donut hole. After spending $5,100, the person exited the donut hole, and coverage kicked back in to cover 95 percent of the cost of drugs. The donut hole was scheduled to change in size with every passing year.

A good way to visualize how the Part D plan works presently is to understand it as a matter of four phases. First is the deductible phase, during which enrollees pay $505 (as of 2022) regardless of whether they purchase any drugs or not. Second, the initial coverage phase, during which enrollees pay 25 percent of the cost of drugs until the total amount they spend reaches $4,430. This is the "true out-of-pocket" cost, or TrOOP, according to Medicare. Third, the coverage gap phase, or donut hole, begins. The coverage gap continues until TrOOP reaches $7,050.

Due to the Affordable Care Act, what enrollees in the donut hole were required to pay was reduced to 25 percent. In order for that to happen, manufacturers were required to contribute. The calculation for phase three is tricky. Medicare explains it this way.

> The drug manufacturer pays 70% of the drug costs, and this counts towards TrOOP. So 95% of drug costs are counting toward TrOOP while in the coverage gap phase, even though the enrollee is only paying 25%. This means that the $7,050 level (in 2022) will be reached after the enrollee has paid $1,469 while in the coverage gap phase. . . . This brings the enrollee's total spending to about $2,937 for the year.[2]

Phase four, the catastrophic phase, begins if and when the enrollee spends enough to exit the donut hole. During the catastrophic phase, enrollees pay 5 percent of drug costs or small copays, whichever is greater. In 2022, the copays were $3.90 for generics and $9.85 for brand-name drugs. The passage of the Inflation Reduction Act of 2022 changed that. Enrollees would no longer be required to pay anything once they reached the catastrophic phase after 2024. While it is true that few people reach the catastrophic phase of the Part D plan, for those who do, this is a major benefit.

I won't ask if you now understand how Part D costs are calculated because we can agree that it's confusing. So, you might think prospective Part D enrollees would find the complications off-putting. Not so. The Medicare administration claims that this is one of its most popular programs. That must be true since 49 million people were enrolled in Part D plans in 2022. It is undoubtedly so popular because people perceive it to be a good deal given how much they would have to pay if they didn't have insurance—the costs of drugs can be astronomical. According to Medicare calculations, the average Part D monthly premium is $31.50. (We will return to pharmaceutical costs in chapter 7.)

PART C—MEDICARE ADVANTAGE PLANS

Part C was known as Medicare + Choice when it was introduced in 1997. Under this arrangement, Medicare was to pay private insurance companies a fixed fee to provide a package of healthcare services, combining Parts A and B. The plan was designed as a capitation arrangement. The number of plans grew to 345 in the first year. When the government looked into who chose to enroll in Medicare + Choice plans a few years later, it discovered that enrollees were generally younger and healthier than the general Medicare population. Moreover, it found that those who did become seriously ill proceeded to drop out of the Part C plans and shift back to traditional Medicare. Given these findings, the Medicare administration determined it was overpaying and proceeded to reduce the rate it offered private insurance companies to provide Medicare + Choice plans. Companies selling the plans responded by increasing how much enrollees would have to pay out-of-pocket.

The rules governing Medicare + Choice were revised in 2003 in conjunction with the passage of Part D, the Medicare Prescription Drug, Improvement, and Modernization Act. The Part C plan was renamed Medicare Advantage. In passing this legislation, the government agreed to pay insurance companies 8.4 percent *more* per Medicare Advantage enrollee than how much it was spending on enrollees in Medicare Part A and B, known as traditional Medicare. Proponents presented it as a cost-containment measure based on the idea that private companies needed an incentive to offer alternatives to government plans. They predicted that the existence of alternative plans would ultimately reduce costs through competition because private companies were sure to introduce efficiency measures and cost-saving innovations. Those predictions were well off the mark. By all accounts, over the next few years, the amount the government was paying private companies over and above the cost of Part A and Part B edged up to 14 percent, reaching a high of 19 percent in some rural areas.

The enrollment period for Medicare Advantage is January 1 through March 31, but it is advertised during the traditional Medicare enrollment period too. You can't miss knowing that Medicare Advantage is available (for about half of the year) if you turn on the television. You can expect to be treated to seeing an enormous number of ads featuring older adults acting absolutely giddy upon hearing that they can sign up for whatever Medicare Advantage plan is being touted.

MEDICARE ADVANTAGE BUSINESS OPERATIONS

Medicare Advantage organizations earn income through a process that starts with a bid reviewed by the Centers for Medicare & Medicaid Services (CMS) in which they agree to cover all the services Medicare covers plus any other services they wish to add, such as dental and vision services. The bid is compared to a *benchmark* set at the rate Medicare pays for fee-for-service Medicare enrollees in the county where the plans expect to operate. Plans with bids below the benchmark get to keep the difference as a rebate.

The ACA created an adjustment to how benchmarks are set in recognition of the fact that the cost of living in some areas of the country is lower than in others, with urban areas generally having higher costs. Plans operating in the counties with a high cost of living receive 95 percent of the county benchmark; those in lowest-cost counties receive 115 percent.

Medicare Advantage plan companies can earn a higher rate of reimbursement based on performance. Plans are rated using a star rating system that assesses care processes, care management, beneficiary satisfaction, and administration. Highly rated plans can see their benchmark increase by up to ten percent.

Plans can also increase the reimbursement they receive if they can show that they are spending more to care for higher-risk patients. They do this through *risk adjustment*. Recognizing the need to adjust payment, Congress instituted higher payments for the care of sicker patients. Critics say that the promise of a higher rate based on risk assessment caused Medicare Advantage plans to engage in "up-coding," that is, making enrollees look sicker than they really are. According to the Medicare Payment Advisory Commission (MedPAC), risk assessments in 2020 were about 9.5 percent higher than what they would have been for a person in traditional Medicare, resulting in about $12 billion in excess payments.[3] In 2021, Medicare Advantage plans were paid $11,844 per enrollee, which is $321 more than Medicare would have paid per enrollee in traditional Medicare.[4] Medicare Advantage plans reported a return of $350 billion that year. Based on the rate of growth in enrollment, that sum is expected to increase to $664 billion by 2029. As the article in which these data are reported states—this presents a challenge to Medicare's solvency.

An expose published by the *New York Times* in 2022 states that a former top health official estimated that overpayments are actually over $25 billion.[5] The story documents whistle-blowers' accounts of physicians being pressured or bribed to submit additional diagnoses. They go on to report the following:

> Eight of the 10 biggest Medicare Advantage insurers—representing more than two thirds of the market—have submitted inflated bills, according to the federal audits. And four of the five largest players, UnitedHealth, Humana, Elevance and Kaiser—have faced federal lawsuits alleging that efforts to overdiagnose their customers crossed the line into fraud.

The authors say that overpayment has been the subject of "inspector general investigations, academic research, Government Accountability Office studies, MedPAC reports, and numerous news articles over the course of four presidential administrations." They conclude by asking the following: Why has CMS been less than aggressive in monitoring these practices?

Medicare Advantage is receiving so much attention because enrollment continues to grow. Part of the explanation is that the baby boom generation entered its golden years in 2011. Although this population is healthier than comparable cohorts in the past, people in this age group are still likely to have two or more chronic diseases. Consider two additional facts: (1) about

76 million people were born between 1946 and 1964; and (2) the number of people over the age of eighty-five is expected to double by 2040.

The steady increase in Medicare Advantage enrollments and mushrooming costs are causing policy analysts to question prevailing policies. One question that keeps coming up is whether tying benchmarks to traditional Medicare expenditures makes sense if those who do not join Medicare Advantage plans are older and sicker, as evidence has shown to be true in the past. The controversies swirling around this issue have escalated over recent years.

Medicare Advantage plans have been both aggressive and inventive in recruiting new enrollees. For example, they have been known to locate enrollment offices in spaces requiring climbing stairs to discourage less healthy patients and offer gym memberships to recruit healthier ones.

Another issue is whether the profits the plans earn are being taxed correctly. Here is the underlying problem. As you will recall, one of the changes the ACA made in how insurance plans operate is that it instituted a *medical-loss ratio* of 15 percent for large group plans and 20 percent for small market plans. According to a Brookings Institution study, health insurance companies now report roughly 5 percent margins (profits), which might be interpreted as an important legislative success. However, the authors of the report question how accurately this captures what Medicare Advantage organizations actually earn, given that they have related businesses not governed by the medical-loss ratio. The five biggest Medicare Advantage plans "all have related businesses including PBMs [Pharmacy Benefit Manager companies], post-acute providers, hospitals, and physician-practices, to name a few. . . . This creates potential to move earnings outside of the reach of regulations."[6]

Other observers worry that enrollment appears to be moving toward a Medicare Advantage-dominated system, which, they say, cannot be expected to work toward the public purposes the Medicare program has served during its lifetime. Medicare has shaped the healthcare system by supporting medical education, setting quality standards, collecting information on care patterns throughout the country, supporting healthcare centers, including rural centers, supporting financing experiments such as Accountable Care Organizations, and so on. They argue, "The Medicare program must also consider how to sustain Medicare's record of innovation in payment and delivery-system reform in a program in which the nature and results of innovation are increasingly the proprietary property of private entities."[7]

Finally, after hearing policymakers' concerns about Medicare Advantage administrative costs and profits, it is worth noting that, in contrast to the medical-loss-ratio Medicare Advantage organizations enjoy, traditional Medicare carries out its administrative responsibilities at the cost of 2 percent of program expenditures.

MEDICAID

Medicaid was the other major public health insurance program legislated in 1965 as an amendment (Title 19) to the Social Security Act. Its first full year of operation was 1967.

Medicaid is a joint federal-state program. The federal government allows states a fair amount of leeway in determining eligibility based on income. States are permitted to set the eligibility cut-off at a percent of the current federal poverty line, well above or well below that line. The 2022 eligibility rates are as follows: the lowest eligibility cut-off is in Texas at 17 percent of poverty and Alabama at 18 percent. At the other end of the continuum, at the high end is Washington, DC, at 251 percent of poverty, with Connecticut next at 155 percent for parents and 138 percent for all others in the state.

The legislation mandates that the federal government accepts responsibility for half of each state's Medicaid outlay, more if the state has an especially high proportion of poor people. This averages out to 56 percent of Medicaid costs across states.

The Medicaid program experienced immense expansion over the years. In 1970, it enrolled 14 million persons and had a budget of $5 billion. By 2020–2021, enrollment had increased to 82.7 million with a budget of $671.2 million. (By comparison, the Medicare program enrolled 63.9 million persons and cost $829.5 billion over this period.)

The Medicaid program evolved over time. Initially, adults without small children were not eligible, no matter how poor. However, the federal government made changes over the years after the law was passed. According to one account, by 2003, Medicaid required states to provide coverage for twenty-eight additional specific categories of people, allowing them to choose to cover up to twenty-one optional eligibility groups.[8] For example, the federal government began requiring coverage for children under the age of eighteen and pregnant women below 133 percent of poverty. While states were not required to cover both parents and children in low-income families, they were permitted to do so.

Unlike Medicare, which was created as an entitlement program, Medicaid was created as a "means-tested" program. Applicants were required to prove that they were poor enough to qualify. Critics of the means testing requirement argued that it was degrading and stigmatizing to have to prove that one is poor. Furthermore, they said that means-testing wasted funds on checking eligibility that could be better spent on the delivery of health care. It's not hard to see why administrative costs would be sizeable, considering how much paperwork and clerical time was required to verify eligibility (think about how many people were needed to do this before computers came on the scene). Furthermore, because applicants' incomes could vary over the year, they had to reapply if their income increased and then fell again. This is known as "churning." The practice has become less common but has not been eliminated.

THE ACA AND REFORM

The Affordable Care Act introduced a number of additional reforms addressed to Medicaid, which did not last. One of the most significant was the expansion of Medicaid to all adults under age sixty-five with incomes under 133 percent of poverty. Adjustments increased this figure to 138 percent of poverty. The ACA provided coverage for adults with no dependent children for the first time in many states.

Governors in some states who stood firmly in opposition to the mandates introduced by the ACA made it clear that they would not extend Medicaid in their states. In fact, days after the law was passed, twenty-six states filed lawsuits challenging the implementation of the ACA. The Supreme Court handed down its ruling challenging the ACA in June 2012, upholding the constitutionality of the body of the law but ruling the Medicaid expansion portion of the law unconstitutional. The governors of states involved in the suit also objected to the requirement that they create state Health Exchanges, that is, marketplaces where people could purchase private insurance. The Supreme Court decision meant that the twenty-six states could keep the Medicaid funding they were already receiving and would not have to expand their Medicaid programs but would have to create Health Exchanges. Quite a few states have reversed their stance on Medicaid expansion since then. As of 2023, ten states continue to refuse to expand Medicaid. This includes Alabama, Florida, Georgia, Kansas, Mississippi, South Carolina, Tennessee, Texas, Wisconsin, and Wyoming, leaving 2.1 million people in the *coverage gap*.

In some cases, governors in states that favored Medicaid expansion were afraid they could not come up with the funds to implement the Medicaid reform. The federal government responded by agreeing to cover 100 percent of the cost of healthcare services for all new enrollees from 2014 through 2016 and 95 percent in 2017, gradually dropping that rate over the following years to 90 percent by 2020.

Income is not the only consideration for Medicaid eligibility. Medicaid eligibility requires a person to prove they have no wealth. The standard wealth cut-off is $2,000, but states can set it higher. There are a few notable exceptions, such as the cut-off in New York state, which is $15,000. The restriction on wealth means she must cash in everything she owns before she can say she is truly impoverished. ("She" is appropriate here because there are more poor elderly women than men; because they outlive men and earn less over their working lives, they have less of a savings cushion.) The person can't own a house or a car worth more than whatever the state decides, and so on. All financial records must be submitted to the state agency that carries out the review.

Consider the implications of Medicaid eligibility for potential enrollees. What if a person has a pension that puts the person above the poverty line but that person runs up such high medical bills that they end up being impoverished with very little money left to live on? This is called the "spend down" provision. A person may become eligible for Medicaid because so much of their money (e.g., social security check and/or pension) goes to paying medical bills.

Medicaid eligibility based on income and wealth comes into question if and when a person seeks to be admitted to a nursing home. Remember, Medicare covers nursing home care for a limited period and only after hospitalization. What about people who require assistance because they are chronically ill, frail, confused, and need help with medications, toileting, eating, and so forth? The determination that the person needs long-term nursing home care in such cases is made by the family, and a period of hospitalization is not necessarily involved. People who are incapacitated enough to go into a nursing home typically give up whatever monies they have to their children, which makes them impoverished and eligible for Medicaid. The only other option is to pay for it out of one's pocket. Given that nursing home care averaged about $10,000 per month for a private room with no added services in 2020, while Medicaid coverage is free if one qualifies for it, you can understand why Medicaid is such an important alternative and is now providing coverage for an increasing number of people in nursing homes.

Medicaid enrollment stood at about 90,000 persons in 2019. The number rose significantly in 2020 when President Biden declared a Public Health Emergency and Congress passed the $15 billion America Rescue Plan Act (ARPA) to extend Medicaid to states that had not adopted the Medicaid extension authorized by the ACA. The legislation added a 5 percent benefit on top of the 90 percent coverage already in effect. The law was in effect through 2022. The Inflation Reduction Act legislated in 2022 extended ARPA subsidies through 2025.

PUBLIC OPINION AND MEDICAID

What accounts for the resistance to Medicaid expansion among states that refused to expand is worth reflecting on. That stance is grounded in the country's long-standing attitudes about persons enrolled in social welfare programs. Critics initially said the Medicaid program was a handout to unde-serving members of society, with most scorn directed toward poor, single mothers. When the program began to cover adult men and women with no children, the new enrollees were labeled malingerers, who, the critics said, would have health insurance if they chose to work but refused to do so. They were portrayed as people who sit around doing nothing productive but some-how manage to eat steak and drive fancy cars. Admittedly that assessment has changed to some extent as increasing numbers of people find that their aged family members need to apply for Medicaid services but not enough to alter the positions taken by politicians in some states.

Consider what happened during the last years of the Trump administration. Trump allowed thirteen states to use Section 1115 demonstration waivers to impose work requirements. The waivers were created to encourage states to come up with innovations that would benefit enrollees. The govern-ment welcomed reductions in program costs, but this was not necessarily the most important objective. Innovative healthcare delivery arrangements were prioritized. Attempts to impose work requirements had been tried but failed at the federal level, and no state had ever received a waiver for this purpose before this time. The Biden administration withdrew approval for the work-requirement clause based on the assessment that the waivers do not promote the objectives of the Medicaid program.[9]

With the charge in mind that Medicaid applicants are undeserving of government assistance, it is essential to recognize that while all enrollees are entitled to use healthcare services, they do not necessarily all seek health care. The picture of who is enrolled and who uses Medicaid services is illuminating.

Table 4.1 makes clear that the categories of recipients responsible for over 50 percent of expenditures are seniors and the disabled. The two original enrollee categories—adults and children—are responsible for just over a quarter of expenditures. Then there's the "newly eligible adults" category. That group consists of persons who suddenly became eligible for Medicaid benefits because of the extension mandated by the ACA. There hasn't been much attention directed to this group, but it is reasonable to assume that these are people who had no health insurance before they became eligible for Medicaid in 2013; and that they had health problems they didn't have the financial resources to deal with before this time, likely making the problems more severe and expensive to treat when they were finally addressed.

Finally, there are those who qualify for both Medicaid and Medicare, the "dual eligibles." In 2019, they numbered 12.2 million and accounted for $440.2 million in expenditures. The dual eligibles are older adults with mul-tiple health problems who may not have started out poor but ended up being poor because of high medical costs. Policy analysts repeatedly point out that

Table 4.1. Medicaid enrollees and recipients, 2019

	% Enrollees	% Recipients
Seniors	10	21
Disabled	11	34
Adults	39	10
Newly eligible adults	22	17
Children	40	17

Source: "Medicaid Spending by Enrollment Group." KFF. 2019. Medicaid Spending by Enrollment Group. https://www.kff.org/medicaid/state-indicator/medicaid-spending-by-enrollment-group/?currentTimeframe =0&sortModel=%7B%22colId%22:%22Location%22,%22sort%22:%22asc%22%7D.

no healthcare system reforms will reduce the costs of treating this population short of the denial of care. This is not a policy anyone has been ready to articulate to date, at least not publicly.

MEDICAID AND MANAGED CARE

The administration of Medicaid programs deserves attention. An increasing number of states have opted to contract with private-sector managed-care organizations, hiring them to handle the provision of healthcare services to their Medicaid enrollees. As of 2022, forty-one states have entered into managed care contracts covering 69 percent of all Medicaid enrollees. States negotiate how much they will pay per person, the capitation rate, and leave the rest to the managed care organization. These organizations must follow rules similar to those governing the Medicare Advantage organizations. They are not coming in for criticism because they have improved access to care for the populations they serve.

STATE CHILD HEALTH INSURANCE PROGRAM

The State Child Health Insurance Program (known initially as SCHIP, now known as CHIP), or Title 21 of the Social Security Act, was legislated in conjunction with the budget reform legislation of 1997. It was passed in response to what everyone who looked at health insurance and poverty data realized at the time: poor and near-poor children were at particularly high risk of being uninsured. The intent was to provide health insurance for children under the age of nineteen whose family income was too high to qualify for Medicaid but too low to allow for the purchase of private health insurance. The funds to cover the program must be reauthorized periodically. CHIP is currently funded through 2028.

Eligibility varies by state from 170 to 400 percent of poverty. States may use one of three options for establishing and administering CHIP: (1) a separate CHIP program, (2) Medicaid expansion, or (3) some combination. To encourage states to offer CHIP, the government covers 70 percent of the states' costs. As of 2022, 9.6 million children were enrolled, bringing the uninsurance rate among children down to 5 percent. CHIP enrollment is generally not reported separately. It is rolled into Medicaid enrollment.

A short-lived phase in the history of CHIP serves to underline the problems associated with having health insurance programs operated by fifty different state-based agencies. When CHIP legislation was passed, Congress appropriated $40 billion over the next ten years. It made the funds immediately available to states that had administrative procedures in place and were already enrolling children. It took some states longer to create such arrangements than anticipated. As a result, much of the allocated funding was not spent during the first year or two. States in a position to create CHIP programs more quickly began applying for and using the unspent funds to cover childless adults. Politicians representing states not ready to apply for the funds sued, claiming to have been deprived of funding to which they were entitled. Congress was forced to deal with the problem of unspent funds. It passed a so-called SCHIP Fix in 2003, which dealt with the distribution of the remaining unspent funds.

Children still are the poorest members of society, which research repeatedly tells us has serious consequences lasting the individual's entire lifetime and consequences for society as a whole. We will touch on this topic again in chapter 9.

CONTINUING POLICY DEBATES

The story about unspent CHIP funds is just one example of the difficulties that plague the country's healthcare arrangements, namely fragmentation. Of course, not everyone would agree that this is a problem. Some would argue that healthcare coverage is a matter of states' rights and there is no problem. At the same time, few opponents are ready to oppose health insurance coverage for everyone, that is, universal coverage, which virtually all economically advanced countries have had in place for a long time. The problem is there is no agreement on how that should be achieved.

On one side of the debate are those who say health is a human right. On the other side are those who say health care is a commodity, like any other commodity purchased in the marketplace. That leads to debate about whether the best way to provide health insurance is through a single-payer plan for which the government is responsible; or whether the private sector is better at providing coverage because it allows for greater choice and is more efficient.

While the argument about which is the better approach is theoretical, a good deal of evidence is available on how such alternatives work based on the experiences of other countries that have embraced some version of one or the other approach—that is a discussion to which we return in chapter 8.

In the meantime, proposals designed to control costs keep appearing. Many are short-lived. And only a small number receive enough attention to merit in-depth analysis. A proposal for reducing Medicare costs that did receive more attention involved raising the Medicare eligibility age from sixty-five to sixty-seven. The age to qualify for Social Security had already been raised and has apparently worked out well, so why not do it in the case of Medicare? A thoughtful analysis was presented in a report issued by the Kaiser Family Foundation Program on Medicare Policy in 2011.[10]

What follows is a summary of that analysis. Raising the eligibility age by two years would have generated an estimated \$7.6 billion in net Medicare savings for the federal government. It would have required a drop in coverage for about 5 million persons in this age bracket. The projected savings would be offset by the \$8.9 billion the federal government would have to spend for those who would then have to be covered by Medicaid, plus the \$7.5 billion that the federal government would be providing in tax credits to those buying insurance through exchanges. There would be a \$7 billion reduction in Medicare premium receipts. The change would shift a \$4.5 billion burden to employers who would still be the primary providers of insurance for those who continued to work. Everyone buying insurance through exchanges, which would now include sixty-five and sixty-six-year-olds, would pay 3 percent more for coverage because of increased chance of illness in the risk pool; Part B enrollees would also pay 3 percent more because younger Medicare recipients would be out of the risk pool; and states would have to spend \$7 billion to provide Medicaid coverage for the new enrollees.

In short, Medicare expenditures would certainly drop. However, costs would not be eliminated; they would be shifted. What does this cautionary tale tell us? The analysts wanted us to understand that cost shifting does not achieve cost savings and may even add to government expenditures.

As already stated, efforts to achieve greater cost control by limiting access to health care for the poor are never-ending. While much of the opposition is about the ethics of limiting health care, some basic facts similar to those we just reviewed about increasing the age of eligibility for Medicare also apply. An overwhelming amount of evidence indicates that cutting health insurance to the poor results in increased costs that show up in other ways. We will spend more time addressing this observation in the final chapter of the book.

In the meantime, one policy change aimed at reducing Medicare costs has been implemented and promises to achieve positive results. The Inflation Reduction Act of 2022 requires Medicare to negotiate with drug companies with the aim of reducing pharmaceutical prices. Medicare was explicitly forbidden to do so when the legislation was passed. However, the cost of drugs has been a significant source of public dissatisfaction, which allowed the government to pass legislation in 2022 allowing Medicare to enter into negotiations over drug pricing—more about this in chapter 7.

Chapter 5

Healthcare Occupations

The number of people involved in the delivery of healthcare services in this country increased dramatically over the last century. By 2022, 14 percent of the population was employed in the health sector. The US Census Bureau identified 459 different health occupations. It goes without saying that we can only focus on a small number of them. A projection issued by the Bureau of Labor Statistics (BLS) indicates that it expects 2.6 million new health sector jobs to be added between 2022 and 2030. That would bring the proportion of the US population working in the health sector up to 16 percent. It is no wonder economists consider the health sector the "driving engine of the economy." And not surprisingly, investors are paying attention, which has had a significant effect on the structure of the healthcare system.

According to the Centers for Medicare and Medicaid Services, the total amount of money the country spent on health care in 2021 was $4.3 trillion. That translates into 18.3 percent of GDP. (This percentage is higher than what was cited in the first chapter when we compared US expenditures to those of other countries due to the lag in updating expenditures across all countries.) A quarter of that total went toward professional services. Thirty-three percent was spent on hospital care. The remainder was spent on long-term care, prescription drugs, and health insurance.

Although the largest number of healthcare workers are nurses, this chapter devotes most attention to physicians because they are the ones primarily responsible for diagnosing and treating patients, which translates into charges.

THE MEDICAL PROFESSION

The medical profession can trace its origins to ancient Greece. As an aside, I might add that those roots are alive and well. This is based on a discussion with my dermatologist. As a classics undergrad, he learned Greek. As a medical student, he discovered that the words describing skin problems employed by ancient Greeks are the same as those used now. With a wicked grin on his face, he told me most of the cures are basically the same too.

The development of the medical profession in this country is grounded in the success achieved by one group of practitioners in a crowded field of practitioners: the allopaths. The field of competitors included hydropaths, who used water to soothe but more often than not aggressively heat up or cool down the body; naturopaths, who used natural herbal preparations in the prevention of disease and treatment of symptoms; homeopaths, who treated "like symptoms with like" to attain stability and bring comfort; chiropractors, who used back manipulation and massage; osteopaths, or DOs (doctors of osteopathy), who subscribe to the idea that the backbone is the body's control center and that its strength is central to good health; and allopaths, who engaged in aggressive interventions, such as bloodletting and use of emetics to induce vomiting, and if they were not successful, simply applied more of the same treatment. However, it was the allopaths who succeeded in laying the foundation for mainstream medicine.

By the beginning of the twentieth century, allopathic medicine had firmly allied itself with science. The other practitioners did not exactly disappear, and some, namely the DOs, were largely absorbed by allopathic, now mainstream, medicine. The rest came to be defined as unscientific and lost ground. Practitioners other than mainstream medical doctors now offer what has become known as "complementary" medicine. The scientific community does not deny that complementary medicine may provide benefits. It is just that the diagnoses and treatments are so individualized that they cannot be standardized or confirmed. What works for one person may not work for another. Moreover, the medications these practitioners rely on are not regulated by the one agency that approves drugs in this country, the Federal Drug Administration (FDA). The result is that, as one investigation after another reveals with considerable fanfare, the amount of active ingredient in such medications may or may not be accurate and may not even be there at all. Yet some people continue to swear by these products, and until a scandal occurs, with reports of injury or death, no one demands that better controls be instituted. And after a while, the whole issue dies down again.

What is it about allopathic medicine that made it scientific? It meant that the explanations and, ultimately, the treatments allopathic medicine offered at the end of the nineteenth century could be substantiated. The allopaths could predict the course of disease with and without treatment. The same was true from one instance or one person to another. They verified their diagnoses by doing autopsies. This allowed doctors to compare the symptoms outlined in the patient's file to the effect on the organs involved. They built up a body of knowledge and learned to apply it. An increasing number of people began to believe in their explanations as evidence of their success began to accumulate.

The larger context of the times when all this was taking place may be worth reflecting on. It happened at about the same time that Americans had suddenly become convinced that science was the way to go in all areas of life. During the first decades of the twentieth century, there was talk about scientific solutions for such unlikely pursuits as housewifery (i.e., housekeeping) and such popular ones (in some circles) as scientific management. The growth of confidence in scientific medicine was not a unique phenomenon but a part of a broader shift in social values and expectations.

MEDICAL SPECIALIZATION

Initially, the majority of doctors, that is, the allopaths (hereafter referred to as doctors or physicians), identified themselves as "physician and surgeon." Relatively few chose to perform major surgery of the kind that required a surgical suite in the hospital.

It was the allopaths who went on to focus on one area of practice. That is, they chose to specialize in treating a particular part of the body. The first specialty to emerge was ophthalmology (i.e., medical and surgical treatment of the eye). One reason is that new and better tools were becoming available during the latter half of the nineteenth century, making it easier to detect abnormalities in the eye. By the late 1800s, small groups of doctors were meeting to discuss their observations about the eye and the new tools they had begun to employ. They were the ones who decided to establish a specialty of their own. Why do that? Was the chance to make more money a primary motivation here? A closer look at how people entered most occupations helps answer that question.

At the turn of the century, a person announced his or her occupation by putting up a sign declaring the kinds of work he (mostly he) was prepared to do. You could claim any occupation you wanted in the city directory, which published a person's occupation in addition to their address. People could, and did, simply pick up, move, and start doing different kinds of work whenever it suited them. This might be surprising, but until the last decades of the nineteenth century, there was strong opposition to all forms of licensure. When the movement to institute licensure took hold in the 1880s, it occurred state by state. Today states continue to control licensure, and a medical license to practice from one state may not be honored in another state.

As an aside, the state can issue licenses for whatever it wants. To illustrate, psychologists are permitted to prescribe medications in five states. The argument supporting this decision is that it extends mental health treatment to more people. The argument against it is that psychologists do not have clinical training in the physiological effects of such medications. Politicians decide which position to endorse.

Returning to ophthalmology, wasn't requiring practitioners to have a medical license sufficient to treat problems affecting the eyes? Yes, but it seems that ophthalmology was a special case. Prospective patients were eager to have some assurance that a practitioner did have the best skills when it came to treating the eye. And practitioners wanted to be able to assure patients that they were, in fact, seeing someone who was well-trained.

Physicians who restricted their practices to treating people's eye problems and met with colleagues to upgrade their knowledge on a regular basis did know more about the eye than anyone else. They were the ones who decided to institute specialty "certification." They set up training programs as well as a qualifying exam for recognizing new practitioners as qualified specialists. Thus, in 1916, ophthalmology became the first certified medical specialty.

You may wonder how other physicians reacted to the emergence of certification in ophthalmology. They were generally pleased, as most reputable doctors were not interested in treating eye problems because it is such a complex organ.

Other areas of specialization followed. However, the majority of doctors continued to identify themselves as "physicians and surgeons" and identify what they did as general practice throughout the first half of the twentieth century.

World War II stands as a significant turning point in the development of specialized medicine. The wartime draft made an impression on doctors. Specialists entered military service as captains, while general practitioners entered as lieutenants. Obviously, with the higher rank of captain came higher pay and other privileges. Not the least of which was the fact that captains were assigned to hospitals away from the battleground while the lieutenants were assigned to field hospitals at the front.

Once the war ended, there was the effect of the GI Bill to consider. One of the big rewards for wartime military service was free education upon return. Many veterans took advantage of this benefit, including those who already had a medical degree (MD). They went on to get more education and training better suited to treating patients who were not war casualties. Some opted for specialty training and went on to take certification exams. Others announced that they were specialists based on the fact that they completed all the requirements and were qualified to take certification tests even if they did not actually take that final step.

Continuing to take a historical perspective, we find that the central feature of life in the United States from the mid-1960s through the early 1970s, in addition to the Vietnam War, anti-war protests, and the civil rights movement, was the increased role that the government was playing in civilian life. The government was funneling considerable sums of money into programs of all kinds—education, housing, and social welfare. Suddenly funds became available to medical schools for research. There was an explosion of scientific knowledge. Medical students were not at all sure that they could learn everything they needed to know. This provided additional impetus for turning to specialization.

In the meantime, with all the emphasis on specialization, general practitioners (GPs) were becoming unhappy. They were paid less than specialists for providing many of the same services. Patients were referring themselves to specialists because they perceived specialists to be more knowledgeable. The GPs decided to make themselves specialists in "family practice." In 1971, family practice became a specialty like any other medical or surgical specialty. Up until this time, medical school graduates were required to complete a one-year internship program to obtain a license to practice granted by the state. After 1971, all medical school graduates were expected to complete residencies lasting at least three years, more to become more highly specialized. In short, as of 1971, there would be no new general practitioners coming out of medical school.

We now refer to physicians engaged in diagnosing illness, providing treatment, recommending surgery if necessary, and monitoring a patient's health as "primary care" practitioners. This includes internists, pediatricians, and family practitioners.

As an aside, it is worth noting that one category of specialists—hospitalists—trains to care for hospitalized patients. They serve as intermediaries between the patient's primary care physician, specialists, and other hospital staff. The hospitalist idea was introduced in the late 1970s, but the label didn't exist until 1996, when it appeared in a *New England Journal of Medicine* article.

In another aside, you might be interested in hearing the origins of surgical specialties. They evolved out of the work performed by barber-surgeons in European monasteries who were needed because monks were required to have shaved heads. Their ability to use sharp instruments led to their dealing with injuries sustained in wars, such as the amputation of limbs, for example. The barber-surgeon guild had as its symbol a red-and-white pole representing a bloody limb wrapped in white gauze. Surgeons and barbers separated by the end of the eighteenth century. Barbers continued to use the symbol, placing it outside their shops to identify the service they were offering.

While there are quite a few important figures credited with discoveries that made a huge difference in the development of the practice of both medicine and surgery, a recent account of the contribution made by William Stewart Halsted is interesting.[1] He is credited, by some, to be the father of surgery in this country. He is said to have revolutionized surgical practice by using

cocaine to anesthetize the surgical site. Because he tested the cocaine on him-
self to confirm its anesthetic properties before using it on patients, he became
addicted. This had the effect of tarnishing his reputation. However, that
did not prevent him from being one of the four founders of Johns Hopkins
University Medical School, which became the model for the reform of medical education in this country, a topic to which we turn next.

THE MEDICAL EDUCATION SYSTEM

As already noted, before the twentieth century, anyone interested in setting
up a medical practice could do so without the need to prove competence.
This permitted a wide range of medical training arrangements, largely based
on apprenticeship. The Association of American Medical Colleges (AAMC),
established in 1876 with the intention of improving the quality of medical
education, attempted to address that. However, the event that led to a dramatic
shift in medical education was not launched by the AAMC. It was the product
of a discussion involving leading members of the AMA and the Carnegie
Foundation. The Carnegie Foundation was (and still is) devoted to improving
education at all levels. The result of these meetings, which occurred in 1907,
was that the Carnegie Foundation took on the task of evaluating the state
of medical education. The person invited to assume responsibility for this
assignment was Abraham Flexner.

Flexner visited all 155 medical schools and training programs in existence
at the time. He was welcomed because the Carnegie Foundation was known
to distribute funds to schools. It was not until 1910, just before the Flexner
Report was due to be released, that it became clear that Flexner was actually
rating the schools. He graded them on a scale of A through F. The schools
to which he had given an "F" closed down even before the report was out.
Others began upgrading immediately. Many did not survive. By 1920, only
eighty-five medical schools were left.

The standard against which Flexner rated all other schools was the Johns
Hopkins Medical School. He used it as a model because it grounded its
coursework in a scientific body of knowledge. It required two years of basic
science courses before the school allowed students to see a patient under the
supervision of a senior doctor. That is obviously an expensive proposition
compared to apprenticeship training. It is easy to see why Johns Hopkins
and medical schools like it were not options for those with limited resources.

The Flexner Report had a number of effects. It eliminated schools he rated
as inferior, which were also the schools that students from low-income families could afford. That had an impact on the composition of the occupation.
It reduced the chances of minority students getting a medical education. It

affected women's medical schools, which lacked the resources needed to upgrade. Few women were seeking medical education in those days, and those who did generally did not come from wealthy families. The smaller number of schools meant that fewer students could be accepted, which, in turn, meant that schools could be more selective. The result was that medical school graduates were, going forward, white, male, and members of a higher social class.

The heightened sensitivity in recent years to the impact of the Flexner Report on medical school enrollment led the AAMC to rename its annual award in 2021. It had been called the Flexner Award. Its new name is Award for Excellence in Medical Education.

The AAMC turned its focus to other concerns over the years. One of its recent concerns focuses on the amount of debt medical students accumulate over four years of medical school, which, in 2022, averaged out to $194,280. That figure should not be surprising given the cost of four years of medical school—averaging between $225,000 and $337,000. The AAMC recommends increased financial support for medical education, as is common in most economically advanced countries. However, the topic to which AAMC has devoted the most attention is its conviction that the United States needs to produce more physicians. Indeed, no other organization is as adamant or energetic in making this argument. It is hard to know the ideal number. Would it help to look at countries to which we compare ourselves to see how many physicians they have (table 5.1)?

Does that suggest to you that we have a shortage of physicians? I would argue the answer is not entirely clear. Maybe we have more providers who are not MDs, that is, nurse practitioners and physician assistants, whose contribution to patient care is not reflected in these figures. Another possibility is that we have a maldistribution of physicians rather than a shortage, which is true of other countries that also struggle with the scarcity of providers willing to locate in isolated, rural areas.

Some observers argue that the bigger problem is the shortage of primary care practitioners or, if you like, an oversupply of specialists. The Covid-19 pandemic brought the issue into sharper focus.

Table 5.1. Physicians per 1,000 persons, 2019

Country	Physicians
Canada	2.4
Japan	2.5
Switzerland	4.3
United Kingdom	5.8
United States	2.6

World Bank. "Physicians (per 1000 people)." https://data.worldbank.org/indicator/SH.MED.PHYS.ZS.

At present, primary care physicians represent only about one-third of the over-all physician workforce recommended by the Council on Graduate Medical Education (COGME) report on Advancing Primary Care . . . A closer look reveals declining trends in U.S. medical graduates choosing family medi-cine—14 to 8 percent among allopathic graduates from 2000 to 2005 and 34 to 29 percent among osteopathic graduates from 2001 to 2008. This decline is further magnified by the looming retirement of one-quarter of the primary care physician workforce and an anticipated increase in demand for primary care physicians as the U.S. population grows larger and older.[2]

Furthermore, we spend more on specialist care "than almost every other high-income country. . . . There is good evidence that areas at the county level that have higher densities or higher proportions of primary care physicians and primary care teams, actually controlling for everything else, have better life expectancy."[3]

THE ORGANIZATION OF MEDICAL PRACTICE

Until a few decades ago, most physicians in this country were in private or fee-for-service practice. According to the AMA, as of 2020, 30 percent of physicians are now hospital employees. Forty-four percent of all physicians consider themselves self-employed—they own their practices. As owners, they are in a position to enter into contracts with hospitals and healthcare systems. The result is their practices are partially or wholly owned by those entities. Thus, according to the AMA, 2022 was the first year fewer than half of physicians worked in a practice wholly owned by physicians. Another way of putting it, according to the AMA, is that 70 percent worked directly or indirectly for a hospital or healthcare system.

Physicians have been turning away from private practice for several very clear reasons. Most newly minted physicians aren't in a position to set up a new practice, which requires renting or buying office space, hiring staff, buying all the equipment setting up a new office requires, and installing electronic recordkeeping systems, while paying off educational debt and paying malpractice premiums. All that without a long line of patients ready and waiting at the door to produce an income. Accepting a salaried position avoids such problems. Physicians in well-established practices have increas-ingly opted to be acquired by hospitals and healthcare systems for many of the same reasons.

This trend has gotten the attention of researchers associated with Kaiser Health News, who find that private equity firms are acquiring an increasing number of physician practices. (Remember, as stated at the beginning of this chapter, this is happening because the health sector is expected to expand, promising continuing high financial returns.) The problem is that consolidation can result in near-monopolies. When too many practices belong to corporate owners, the result is "higher prices and diminished quality of care." This is reflected in the fact that "private equity firms have agreed to pay fines of more than $500 million since 2014 to settle at least thirty-four lawsuits filed under the False Claims Act, a federal law that punishes false billing submissions to the federal government with fines."[4]

HOW PHYSICIANS GET PAID

The Medicare payment schedule dominates reimbursement arrangements. Other third-party payers base their payment schedules on it. Medicaid generally pays less; private health insurance plans generally pay more. The Medicare payment schedule is updated annually.

What physicians interested in finding out how much Medicare will reimburse them requires readiness to deal with complexity. The AMA has made the CMS rules explicit, presenting them under the title: "2023 Medicare Physician Payment Schedule Final Rule."

The AMA explanation is as follows: "The formula for calculating payment schedule amounts entails adjusting RUVs, which correspond to services, by the GPCIs, which correspond to payment localities."

According to the CMS, the "payment schedule's impact on a physician's Medicare payments is primarily a function of 3 key factors: (1) the resource-based relative value scale (RBRVS), (2) the geographic practice cost indexes (GPCI), and (3) the monetary conversion factor. The AMA further clarifies how this is calculated by presenting the following two equations."[5]

1. Calculating Total RVU:

   Work RUV* × Work GPCI** + Practice Expense (PE) RVU × PE GPCI + Malpractice (PLI) RVU × PLI GPCI = Total RVU

   *The 2023 physician work, practice expenses, and malpractice RVUs may be found in *Medicare RBRVS: The Physicians' Guide.*
   ** The geographic practice cost indexes (GPCIs) for calendar year (CY) 2023 may also be found in the *Medicare RBRVS: The Physicians' Guide.*
2. Calculating Medicare Payment:

   Total RVU × The CYI 2021 Conversion Factor of $34.6062 (Jan. 1–Dec. 31, 2023) = Medicare Payment

In order to understand any part of these equations, prepare to be buried in more difficult-to-unravel detail. If you decide the formulas are too complicated to work through, I assure you—you aren't alone. Physicians agree.

The origins of the factors used in the formulas date back to the team of economists from Harvard University who, in consultation with the AMA and various interested parties, set about working out a formula for paying physicians in 1992. It took four years. The product was called the Resource Based Relative Value Scale (RBRVS). RUVs, relative value units, are the basic components of the RBRVS. The schedule established a fee for every procedure that doctors perform as defined by the Current Procedural Terminology Code (CPT), which the AMA oversees.

The AMA developed the CPT code for medical records, statistical data collection, and insurance purposes in 1966. It went through several revisions before the CMS adopted it in 1983. It is updated annually by the AMA CPT Editorial Panel, which is, in turn, authorized by the AMA Board of Trustees. The panel is comprised of seventeen members; eleven representatives of medical specialty societies; four representatives nominated by the Blue Cross-Blue Shield Association, the American Association of Health Insurance Plans, the American Hospital Association, and the CMS, respectively; two seats are held by the CPT Health Care Professional Advisory Committee (HCPAC).

. CMS uses the CPT recommendation to create and publish the Medicare Physician Fee Schedule (MedPAC). It covers about 10,000 physician services.

As an aside, this committee has come under criticism regarding its composition over the years from within the ranks of the profession. Primary care practitioners have on occasion complained that the specialty societies dominate, which has the effect of undervaluing the primary care providers' contribution to patient care and underpaying them. However, the committee's composition has not changed since it was established.

The process worked as follows until 2015. The Medicare Payment Advisory Committee (MPAC) gave its recommendation to CMS, which published the result. That involved an interesting glitch having to do with the Sustainable Growth Rate legislation passed in 1997, intended to tie the annual increase in Medicare funding to the annual increase in national productivity. Its purpose was to slow the Medicare rate of growth. But medical practice costs were rising faster than the economy was growing, and the Medicare reimbursement rate was not keeping up. This meant that physician reimbursement dropped as the cost of living rose faster than the reimbursement rate. Congress proceeded to address the problem by passing "doc-fix" legislation every year for seventeen years. That practice ended in 2015. This was when Congress legislated a major revision in how physicians would be paid. It passed the Medicare Access and CHIP Reauthorization Act (MACRA), requiring CMS to implement the Quality Payment Program, an incentive program with two tracks.

Under MACRA, physicians must choose to be paid either through the Merit-based Incentive Payment System (MIPS) or the Alternative Payment Model (APM). The APM model is available to those affiliated with new kinds of organizations, such as Accountable Care Organizations (ACOs), which agree to accept incentive reimbursement arrangements. APM is intended to move physicians into arrangements geared to not only improve quality but "incentivize them to accept increased risk of financial loss" if the organization's costs exceed projections. The objective is to move reimbursement arrangements from "volume to value."

Being paid through a MIPS arrangement requires physicians to report the care they provide based on specific indicators, each of which has its own measures. A physician who chooses this arrangement must identify, track, and report on the following indicators.

1. Quality: constitutes 30 percent of the reimbursement calculation. This indicator has ten measures used to track actions.
2. Improvement activities: 15 percent of the score. This involves another set of measures.
3. Promoting interoperability: 25 percent of the score. This is based on integrating electronic health record technology.
4. Cost: 30 percent of the score. CMS does this calculation based on Medicare reimbursement records.

As you might expect, figuring out how to accommodate these expectations has not been easy for physicians, regardless of whether they choose the MIPS or APM track. MIPS requires individual practitioners to invest time to educate themselves in the process they need to employ to collect the required information. The APM does much of the tracking for physicians associated with organizations that agree to work under an APM contract. Reports of APM organizations struggling and failing were widespread initially. There were no models to follow. The learning process continues. Observations presented in the 2022 article in the *Medical Economics* journal capture the ongoing challenge.

> The trend toward VBC [value-based health care] is clear. Yet transitioning from a volume-based transactional billing model to one that incorporates financial risk and rewards tied to the patient's health outcome is not easy. Successful

implementation of value-based programs requires PCPs [primary care physicians] and physician groups to deploy technologies that provide complex hierarchy support for contract model, onboarding, data capture, digitization, value-based payments and exchange.[6]

In short, the effect of this legislation is profound. While it is true that the independent practitioner was rapidly disappearing before the advent of value-based reimbursement, the introduction of these reimbursement arrangements has accelerated the process of eliminating fee-for-service practice along with the independent practitioner.

MEDICAL PROFESSIONALISM

In the early years of the twentieth century, physicians worked hard to become the model "profession" that many other occupations made every effort to emulate in an attempt to gain some of the privileges associated with this designation. In the case of physicians, this meant respect, trust, high income, access to personal information related to illness, and access to the body. The central feature of medical professionalism was the understanding that the physician would be directly responsible to the patient rather than to some third party standing between doctor and patient. This was firmly embedded in the fee-for-service, private practice arrangement. The AMA and its state affiliates were adamant about it. The AMA did not object to medical faculty taking salaried positions because they were primarily engaged in research rather than patient care. The move toward salaried practice or practices owned by hospitals or health systems has erased references to professionalism.

On the one hand, the shift from fee-for-service practice means that physicians do not have to deal with the business side of managing an office, which is something those who embraced medical professionalism chose not to emphasize. In theory, doctors can now devote themselves to practicing medicine, precisely what they spent years learning to do. On the other hand, employee status or employee-like status means having a boss who not only determines salary and sets work hours but imposes various efficiency measures, like the number of minutes the physician can spend with each patient, which unquestionably infringes on professional autonomy.

It is worth noting that physicians in private practice, who stood as model professionals for so long, were, for legal purposes, considered small business persons, which prevented them from joining together to bargain collectively. They were required to do so on an individual basis or as members of an organization established as a corporate entity. Will the shift in employment status change how they see themselves and their ability to negotiate wages and benefits with increasingly larger and more powerful healthcare organizations?

Or they might opt for a different resolution. If the pressure to be more efficient and produce value for the parent organizations employing them was not enough to cause physicians to band together to register frustration with their work arrangements, the onset of Covid-19 made the situation all that much worse. How did physicians respond? A Mayo Clinic study "found that burnout, workload, fear of infection, anxiety, or depression due to COVID-19 and the number of years in practice were associated with intent to reduce work hours or leave."[7]

A physician writing an editorial in the *New York Times* says it's more than that. He presents a devastating critique of the healthcare system, charging it with responsibility for thousands of preventable deaths due to underinvestment in public health systems and hospitals. He maintains the billing system created by the AMA serves to protect for-profit health care. He ends by saying doctors are leaving medical practice because they can no longer ignore their sense of complicity in putting profits over people.[8] (For a more extended discussion of putting profits over people, see: J. Salmon and S. Thompson, *The Corporatization of American Health Care.*[9])

Demographic trends, specifically an aging population, mean the demand for healthcare services will increase. If one in five physicians who say they plan to leave practice over the next couple of years actually does so, how might things change? Will physician scarcity give them a greater voice in how medical practice is structured? Or will the problem be addressed by the new class of private equity owners of physician practices turning to well-established methods for dealing with "a labor shortage"? That remains to be seen.

MEDICAL ERROR AND MALPRACTICE

The matter of medical error came to public attention in 1999 when the Institute of Medicine (IOM) reported that 44,000 to 98,000 people die in hospitals annually due to preventable errors. While the numbers were actively disputed, everyone agreed that error reduction was a highly laudable objective.

The IOM report clearly stated that the error rate was due to systemic failure in hospitals rather than malpractice by individual doctors. However, the public media chose to focus on individuals, mainly doctors, rather than systemic failure in covering the report, which may have prompted some patients to sue. However, a number of other factors contributed to the medical malpractice crisis that occurred in the late 1990s and early 2000s. Actuarial projections did not account for regulatory changes, which caused insurers to increase the premiums they charged. Managed care was on the rise, which caused physicians in high-risk specialties, such as obstetrics, to shop for lower malpractice premiums, which turned out to be "less reliable and comprehensive."

At about the same time, there were stories in various medical and legal publications documenting giant "pain and suffering" awards decided by juries based on the likeability or attractiveness of the litigant. Many states, starting with California, passed tort reform limiting "pain and suffering" awards. California set the limit at $250,000. Such awards are unrelated to the amount of money courts award to cover other costs, including the cost of caring for the injured party and lost income.

Healthcare systems responded by instituting risk management departments tasked with preventing malpractice events before they happened and dealing with them if and when they did happen. The medical malpractice crisis subsided.

There was some fear of another malpractice crisis brought on by Covid-19.

> The US may be in a lull before an approaching storm of medical liability, which may include unexpected injuries, novel legal claims, rising insurance premiums, and insurers withdrawing from malpractice markets. Covid-19 involves severely ill patients, poorly understood patterns of infection, changing standards of care, hospitals operating at or near capacity, workforces under stress, and the potential or tacit rationing of scarce resources.[10]

After painting this menacing scenario, the authors end by saying, "Whether the US enters another true crisis of availability or affordability of malpractice insurance cannot yet be known."

Well, it's now several years later, and the storm hasn't come. Why dwell on the possibility if it is no longer likely? I would suggest that it is worth reflecting on the problems that authors say need to be addressed to recognize how complicated our healthcare arrangements are, with particular attention to the critical role physicians play in managing to provide healthcare services in the midst of what appears to be a state of turmoil brought on by a pandemic that the healthcare system was not prepared for. At least two significant issues associated with malpractice require attention. For one, there is no reliable count of the number of malpractice suits filed yearly, their outcome, or the amounts that were awarded. A second, more controversial issue involves continuing debate about how malpractice lawyers are paid. They are permitted to accept cases on *contingency*, meaning they are paid only if they win and are paid nothing if they lose. Lawyers say that this allows people who could not afford to hire a lawyer and pay all the costs involved in a trial to be represented. Physicians argue that lawyers are motivated to sue even when there is no evidence of error on the chance of collecting one-third of the settlement if they go to court and win and one-fourth if the case is settled out of court. This practice is considered unethical, and in some cases illegal, in most economically advanced countries.

NURSES

Nursing is the single biggest occupational category in the health sector. In 2021, the Bureau of Labor Statistics (BLS) reported 3,047,530 nurses in the country. Most nurses work in general and surgical hospitals (31 percent) or specialty and psychiatric hospitals (32 percent). The remainder are employed in outpatient clinics (15 percent), home health care (11.5 percent), and doctors' offices (7.5 percent).

Nursing provides an interesting contrast to medicine because it has traditionally been an overwhelmingly female occupation and because its origins are very different than that of doctors. The history of nursing is heavily influenced by the traditions introduced by Florence Nightingale. Before her work during the Crimean War in the 1880s, nursing was not considered a respectable activity for women from good families. It was considered dirty work. Nightingale emphasized the use of skills available to every middle-class young woman, namely, cleaning wounds, changing bandages, and comforting patients. She gained acceptance for nursing as a suitable occupation for a young woman from a respectable family by assuring doctors that nurses were there to assist them and not get in their way. To some extent, that is the problem that nursing has faced ever since.

As hospitals began caring for more seriously ill patients and nurses began working in hospitals, it became clear nurses needed more training. However, nurses' training continued to reflect the philosophy introduced by Nightingale. Nursing schools were opened by hospitals providing on-the-job training rather than education with a theoretical base. Nursing students were expected to live in a dorm with strict rules, to be chaperoned, and to perform nursing tasks in the hospital under supervision for three years. Upon graduation, they received a diploma and were qualified to take a state licensing exam leading to the registered nurse (RN) designation.

At some point, colleges began instituting bachelor's degrees in nursing. After completing four years of college and successfully passing the state licensure exam, a nursing student became an RN, just like the diploma graduate. During the 1960s, when the need for more nurses became more urgent, two-year associate-degree nursing programs were created. The graduates of those programs also became RNs. There were now three different routes into nursing based on varying levels of education and experience. In other words, nursing, as an occupation, did not establish control over the educational system and entry into the occupation. More troubling was that the content of nursing programs varied across the three entry routes. However, since hospitals were their primary employers, the fate of nursing as an occupation was tied to how hospitals decided to treat them.

Anytime hospitals faced a shortage of nurses, hospital administrators did not address the problem by raising nursing salaries, as would happen in most other occupational sectors. They just recruited more student nurses into their diploma programs. At some point during the 1970s, most hospitals closed down their diploma programs as they realized that on-the-job training was not enough to prepare nurses to care for the more seriously ill patients being admitted to hospitals. This did not benefit nursing as much as one might expect because hospitals simply began training other kinds of workers to do specific tasks and aggressively recruiting nurses from other countries.

Because nursing has traditionally been a female occupation, nurses have historically been employees rather than independent practitioners like doctors, and their training does not take nearly as long as medical school, which are factors that explain nursing's occupational fate.

At the same time, the unremitting shortage of nurses constitutes a continuing problem. It means that nurses are often required to work more hours than they signed on for. They respond by periodically engaging in organized protests aimed at addressing workload, which they maintain has a direct impact on the quality of care they can deliver. They argue that being overworked and overstressed risks causing them to make errors in patient care.

California was the first state to pass a statute requiring hospitals to maintain an eight-to-one patient-to-nursing staff ratio in 2003 and a three-to-one ratio in the intensive care unit (ICU). The conventional wisdom says that what happens in California predicts what will be happening in other parts of the country in the future. That is certainly true in this case. The battle was successfully waged by the California Nurses Association (CNA), which split off from the American Nurses Association (ANA). In 2009, the CNA joined the Massachusetts Nurses Association and United American Nurses, a unit within the American Nurses Association, to form National Nurses United (NNU), the largest nurses' union in the country. Nursing strikes across the country continue as more nurses quit in response to being exhausted by their experience with Covid. Those who remain say they are being pressed into taking on responsibility for more patients than they can handle.

Nursing embraces professionalism to the extent that it has worked to carve out niches in which nurses can work more independently. Various "advanced practice" nursing programs have come into existence, including nurse-midwifery (delivering babies), nurse anesthetist programs, and nurse practitioner programs. Nurse practitioners and certified nurse midwives serve as primary healthcare providers in underserved areas. This requires master's degree–level training. There are doctoral-level programs leading to a PhD or doctorate in nursing practice.

Nurse midwives also work with doctors to manage normal pregnancies in urban and suburban communities. Studies regularly show that women are very satisfied with the care they receive from nurse midwives. There seems to be no difference in birth outcomes between deliveries managed by nurse midwives and doctors, which may be because nurse midwives are willing to refer high-risk pregnancies to doctors.

Nurses with advanced degrees who work in hospitals typically have managerial responsibilities in addition to patient care responsibilities. They oversee the work of RNs and licensed practical nurses (LPNs), who receive anywhere from six months to over a year of training; nursing assistants who receive certification with 160 hours of training; and unit clerks who are hired without special training to carry out the secretarial tasks for nurses in a hospital.

THERAPISTS

A wide range of occupational groups falls under this designation. Two of the most commonly recognized are physical therapists and occupational therapists. Activities therapists (in music or art) work with patients hospitalized for extended stays. Then there are all the other categories of therapists who work in hospitals, such as respiratory therapists.

Audiologists and speech therapists work in hospitals but may also have private offices and private practices. In addition, some other occupational groups doing psychological counseling consider themselves therapists. In short, therapists come to this work from wide-ranging backgrounds and with a variety of degrees.

TECHNICIANS AND TECHNOLOGISTS

Technicians constitute an even broader category. Medical technicians work in hospitals or outpatient clinics and laboratories. X-ray technicians work directly with patients and have been around for a long time. However, there are now technicians associated with all kinds of diagnostic equipment whose work is similar to that of X-ray technicians, for example, sonography technicians, CT technicians, mammography technologists, nuclear medicine technologists, and so on. Many new occupational categories came on board in hospitals as hospitals created new jobs and trained people to do particular tasks. Hospitals were primarily responsible for training pharmacy technicians to count pills and bottle them, blood technicians to draw patients' blood, and so on.

Physicians' assistants (PAs) don't fit neatly into any designations identified so far. According to the American Academy of Physician Assistants (AAPA), 148,560 certified PAs work in the field. Their ranks increased by 28.6 percent between 2016 and 2020. They differ from nurse practitioners in that PAs work under the physician's license, while nurse practitioners work under their own licenses. There is a movement to change the name from "physician assistant" to "physician associate," which some physicians agree more accurately reflects the work these people do.

Then there are emergency medical technicians (EMTs). They attend to people in an ambulance in an emergency. Their job is to stabilize patients and get them to the emergency room. In some ways, their work is comparable to that of physicians' assistants in that they take direct responsibility for the patient under the guidance of a physician. EMTs connect patients to equipment that emergency room physicians monitor. But it is the EMTs who administer treatment.

OTHER PRACTITIONERS

There are two categories of practitioners known as "limited practice" doctors. This includes podiatrists, who are licensed to treat the full range of foot ailments, and dentists, who treat teeth and gums. Dentists and podiatrists are licensed to perform surgery and administer medications. These privileges differentiate them from other practitioners, who may also call themselves doctors but who do not have such privileges. An example is optometrists, who are licensed to examine the eye and prescribe lenses but must refer patients to an ophthalmologist when they detect eye disease.

Pharmacists are licensed to dispense medications but not prescribe them, even though, in many instances, they know a great deal more about drug interactions than doctors do. In some teaching hospitals, clinical pharmacists with advanced degrees go on "rounds" together with medical staff to explain drug interactions to medical residents.

ADMINISTRATORS AND OTHER
ADMINISTRATIVE WORKERS

Hospital administrators generally come to this work with master's degrees in hospital administration or a comparable degree. The degrees are granted by business schools, schools of public health, medical schools, and various other kinds of programs. The coursework is, however, not all that different. They are also employed in other healthcare delivery settings, including extended care facilities, outpatient facilities, managed care settings, and psychiatric hospitals.

The scope of their responsibility is interesting to consider. Their authority comes from the hospital board of directors or the board of trustees, depending on whether the institution is for-profit or nonprofit. They have responsibility for the organization on a day-to-day basis. Decisions involving financial expenditures are the province of the board.

One of their most significant responsibilities involves overseeing record-keeping. And as we have seen, there are records of all kinds, starting with those that any organization must handle, such as payroll and purchasing. Far more complicated are all the electronic records required by the government and other third-party payers. And as you know, hospitals rely on such reports to bill third-party payers for the goods and services they provide.

Hospital medical records departments, where medical records technicians work, have been one of the fastest-growing occupational areas in the health sector because of the vast amount of information that must be recorded. And it has changed dramatically. Until the last couple of decades of the twentieth century, medical recordkeeping was a matter of filing pieces of paper. It's been a matter of keeping computerized records for some time. Learning to code for the goods and services that physicians and hospitals provide requires training offered by various organizations.

We turn to hospital billing and patient recordkeeping arrangements next.

Chapter 6

Hospitals and Other Healthcare Organizations

When hospitals were inundated with an unprecedented number of very sick, highly infectious patients from early 2020 through the spring of 2022, we could not avoid hearing about it. The news media gave us a running account. We were told we shouldn't go to the emergency room if we could avoid it because ERs were packed with people suffering from Covid. We heard hospitals were canceling scheduled procedures because there were no empty beds. Interviews with doctors and nurses indicated they were working overtime to cover for sick colleagues. They said they were exhausted and overwhelmed—they looked it too. We kept hearing how close to collapsing hospitals were during that period.

As we all know, by the summer of 2022, things finally seemed to settle down. Fewer people were hospitalized for Covid because the virus had mutated into a more infectious but less lethal strain. And the news media turned its attention to new crises. The unstated message was that problems facing hospitals were something the public need not be concerned about any longer. Health policy experts were not nearly as ready to move on. They wanted to understand better how the hospital sector performed at the height of the crisis and whether hospitals were planning to make any changes in response to what they had experienced.

Here's what we've learned since then. For a start, it did not take long for health policy analysts to come out with strong assertions about hospitals needing to be better prepared for the next epidemic. In assessing hospital performance, the analysts pointed out that the country devotes an enormous amount of money to hospitals and that this was the right time to look into where it was all going. Remember, we spent about $4.3 *trillion*, or 18.3 percent of GDP, on health care in 2021. Over 30 percent of the total went to the hospital sector.

To understand what makes hospital care cost so much, we need to have a better appreciation of the hospital sector as a whole. Let's start with three big-picture hospital characteristics. One fundamental characteristic is *length of stay*. Hospitals are either *short-term stay*, *acute care* hospitals, or *long-term stay* hospitals. Long-term stay hospitals generally provide inpatient mental healthcare or rehabilitation services. Nursing homes are the largest category of long-term care facilities. Unless otherwise indicated, the discussion to follow refers to short-term acute care hospitals.

Size is another meaningful characteristic. There are various ways to measure size, including the number of employees, annual budget, kinds of specialty units, number of branches, and so on. The commonly agreed-upon measure of size is the number of beds. A hospital in a rural area might have as few as twenty-five beds, while an urban medical center hospital can have 900 beds. Even though we spend far more on health care than other economically advanced countries, we have fewer hospital beds, at 2.6 beds per 1,000 people. There is some variation in the number of beds reported by the other countries to which we compare ourselves. Some countries have many more, but most have close to the US number. At the high end, Japan has thirteen beds per 1,000 persons, and Germany has eight beds per 1,000 persons.[1] The number of hospital beds a country has does not seem to be closely related to the health status of the country's population.

Hospital ownership is the third major differentiating characteristic. When the government reports hospital statistics, it begins by distinguishing between those owned by the federal government and all other hospitals. Federally owned hospitals are either the Veterans Administration (VA) hospitals operating for the exclusive use of veterans or military hospitals used by active members of the armed forces. Now and then, we hear about the work one hospital the federal government operates, the National Institutes of Health (NIH) Clinical Center, located in Bethesda, Maryland. It is the largest hospital in the country devoted to clinical research, with 1,600 research studies currently being conducted.

Nonfederal hospitals are divided into three ownership categories: (1) nonprofit, (2) for-profit, and (3) state-local government. Hospitals in the state and local government category are the easiest to recognize. They are often named to indicate that they are government-sponsored, like Boston City Hospital, Los Angeles County Hospital, or University of Illinois Hospital. The state and local government hospitals are, in the broadest sense, not-for-profit organizations. Such hospitals are typically referred to as *public* hospitals, meaning they are supported by the public through state or local taxes.

All other hospitals are "community" hospitals. The majority were established years ago as *nonprofit* entities by religious orders, groups aiming to provide for the healthcare needs of their own religious or ethnic group, or by residents of a particular geographic community.

Some were established by individuals, typically one or more doctors. As owners, they made all the decisions on the need for improvements, additional staff, and so on. They pocketed what they earned from running the hospital and paid taxes on their earnings. That made these establishments *for-profit* organizations. They were largely indistinguishable from community non-profit hospitals until well into the second half of the twentieth century. As founders died out and corporate entities took over, for-profit hospitals became known as investor-owned hospitals.

The mix of hospitals has changed over time. The government published the first count of hospitals in 1975.

A number of trends are readily apparent in table 6.1, starting with the drop in the total number of hospitals over time. The only category experiencing growth is the for-profit sector. However, the largest number of hospitals and hospital beds have consistently been in the nonprofit sector. Before we get to what accounts for these trends, let's go back to the beginning of the twentieth century to see how hospitals evolved.

A BRIEF HISTORY OF THE MODERN HOSPITAL

Before the twentieth century, hospitals in this country and elsewhere were primarily charitable institutions established to house people who had no one to look after them. Exactly how many hospitals there were in this country at any point in history is not clear. According to one of the earliest estimates available, there were 178 as of the mid-1880s.[2] Patients admitted to hospitals during that era were invariably poor, some at an advanced stage of disease.

Table 6.1. US hospitals by type and size, 1975–2015

	Number of Hospitals in the United States		Number of Hospital Beds in the United States	
	1975*	2022*	1975*	2015**
All Hospitals	7,150	6,093	1,465,828	897,961
Federal	359	207	131,946	38,863
Community				
Nonprofit	3,322	2,960	658,195	530,579
For-profit	730	1,228	73,495	134,569
State-local	1,778	951	210,154	117,040

*Table 89. "Hospitals, beds, and occupancy rates, by type of ownership and size of hospital: United States, selected years 1975–2015." Health United States. 2017.

** "Fast Facts on U.S. Hospitals, 2022." AHA Hospital Statistics. 2022.

Physicians were willing to volunteer their services in charity hospitals to treat such patients for free because the patients served as interesting "clinical material."

While most people would not have chosen to go to a hospital at the beginning of the twentieth century, surgeons began to find it difficult to perform surgery outside of a hospital operating room. They had started to perform more invasive surgery due to various technological advances. Anesthesia, although not particularly reliable or effective, was introduced in the 1840s. (Imagine what surgery was like before anesthesia. People died even before they had a chance to develop an infection; if they survived, infection was highly likely.) Antisepsis (a sterile surgical environment) had become a regular feature of the surgical suite as of the 1860s. X-ray technology came into existence in the 1890s.

Surgeons did begin to admit middle-class patients during the first decades of the twentieth century who agreed to be admitted only if they could be assured of a clean and safe environment for which they were ready to pay. Hospitals were eager to accept paying patients. Surgeons, in a position to funnel their paying patients to the hospital of their choice, demanded improvements in the quality of surgical suites, equipment, and staff. Hospitals were left with little alternative but to accede to those demands.

Surgeons interested in promoting quality of care came together to form the American College of Surgeons (ACS) in 1913. Physicians established the American College of Physicians (ACP) in 1915 for similar reasons.

One of the primary objectives of these professional associations was to ensure that their colleagues were well-qualified and that the hospitals with which they were affiliated were well-equipped and well-managed. The mechanism prominent physicians adopted to advance the quality of care was the autopsy. It provided an opportunity for doctors to discuss cases and advance medical knowledge. The public nature of the autopsy helped to ensure that the privileges of doctors misdiagnosing patients or doing inappropriate surgeries would be restricted. In short, physicians and surgeons took steps aimed at establishing firm control over the day-to-day activities taking place in hospitals.

Hospital directors, known as superintendents, were well aware of the fact that their interests were not identical to those of surgeons and physicians. They had organized themselves into an association of their own in 1899, the Association of Hospital Superintendents of the United States and Canada. It became the American Hospital Association (AHA) in 1906. Superintendents became known as hospital administrators.

AHA members generally agreed that raising hospital standards was necessary. However, they did not have the power or the resources to achieve that. The AHA first approached the ACS around 1950 to explore the possibility of setting up a cooperative inspection program. Five organizations joined together to develop hospital accreditation standards: the AHA, ACS, ACP, the American Medical Association (AMA), and the Canadian Medical Association (CMA). They worked out standards over the following year and went on to establish a new organization, the Joint Commission on Hospital Accreditation, to carry out the inspections. The inspections were to be carried out voluntarily. Hospitals would have to request them and be charged for carrying them out. It became the Joint Commission on Accreditation of Healthcare Organizations (JCAHO) in 1987 and has, since then, been referred to as the Joint Commission. Other accrediting organizations have come into existence since then, but the Joint Commission is the most well-known. The Joint Commission went on to develop an international division, which is proud to assert that it has awarded its "Gold Seal of Approval" to more than 1,000 healthcare organizations in countries worldwide.

The number of hospitals increased over the first few decades of the twentieth century.[3] According to one of the first AMA counts, there were approximately 4,300 hospitals in the country in 1928. Then the trend suddenly reversed. The drop occurred because of the Great Depression when many people lost their jobs and could not afford hospitalization; those who were taken to one because of an emergency could not pay for it. As a result, many smaller hospitals did not survive. The hospitals that did survive could absorb such losses only because they received contributions from especially dedicated, wealthy contributors. Some hospitals survived because of the support they received from religious orders or the local ethnic community. The only other hospitals that survived the depression were public hospitals.

The hospital sector changed little between the Great Depression and the end of World War II. However, once the war ended, the country experienced a period of adjustment that brought with it not only peace but a period of unprecedented prosperity. It also brought on a housing expansion into newly developing suburban communities, many of which felt they needed a hospital of their own. That brought the Hill–Burton Act into existence in 1946. The federal government matched the funds raised by new communities for the purpose of building a new hospital and by settled communities for adding on to an existing one.

Something besides the objective need for more hospitals may have been involved to explain the urge to build new hospitals and expand old ones. It was evident that many hospitals had come into existence for symbolic reasons. They stood as a major source of community pride, whether ethnic, religious, or geographic. The Hill–Burton Act provided the perfect opportunity to act on that sense of pride. It is also true that some hospitals were built by people who had good reason to believe they were not welcome in hospitals operated by other groups, such as African-American doctors, for a start. Jewish doctors also experienced discrimination when seeking privileges in hospitals run by others. Jewish and African-American patients felt better being treated by doctors who they felt would understand their cultural values. Similarly, Catholic hospitals offered the assurance that patients could practice their religion and that priests would be readily available to offer solace, hear confession, and offer last rites. Immigrants were concerned about being able to communicate and wanted to speak their own language in the hospital. Finally, the newly established suburban communities were interested in proving that they could offer everything the city could offer, only newer and better. In other words, the people building hospitals were certain there was a need for all those new hospitals and new additions—perhaps not the kind of need that policy analysts might be looking for, but "need" in this case was in the eyes of the beholder.

It goes without saying that poor communities could not, and did not, take advantage of the Hill–Burton funds. For this reason, new hospitals were not built in many communities that really needed them. The distribution of hospitals did not get better. As the initial benefactors moved away from some neighborhoods and other, often poorer, people moved in, hospital support systems faltered, and the hospitals closed down.

As an aside, one might ask—why has there been so little effort devoted to planning the distribution of hospitals to reflect need? The answer deserves reflection. The organization of the hospital sector, as it stands at present, is grounded in a fundamental cultural understanding that market forces will prevail. These days, neither religious orders nor nonprofit groups are establishing hospitals in this country. The unstated expectation is that the supply of hospital beds will increase in response to demand. Under these circumstances, the need for a new facility is determined by who is willing to pay to build it and whether there are enough consumers ready to pay for the services it provides.

Getting back to factors responsible for post–World War II hospital expansion, advances in infection control during the late 1940s played a significant role. That is when synthesized penicillin came into existence, becoming widely available by 1950. This was the first time hospitals could control infection with certainty. Newer and more powerful antibiotics followed. It is also true that, over time, the bacteria vexing hospitals grew more powerful. By the end of the twentieth century, hospitals found themselves dealing with "superbugs," such as *Methicillin-resistant Staphylococcus aureus* (MRSA) and *Clostridium difficile* (C. diff). While infection control is a major priority in hospitals, the medical community determined that sending patients home sooner rather than later was the most effective infection-control mechanism available.

GROWTH AND DEVELOPMENT

The fate of the hospital sector is closely linked to the emergence and expansion of health insurance coverage. As you know, the Blue Cross plan established by the Baylor University Hospital in Dallas in 1929 launched employer-based health insurance, increasing the number of people who could afford to be hospitalized. And the postwar economic boom, which brought about Medicare and Medicaid legislation in 1965, caused even more people to seek hospital care.

Health policy experts had reasoned that the backlog of untreated illness would push up Medicare and Medicaid costs initially but that costs would drop once the backlog was reduced. Instead, the plans brought a huge increase in the number of paying patients to hospitals. Rather than dropping, hospital costs rose and continued to climb. Hospitals realized that Medicare, and to a lesser extent Medicaid, plus expansion of private insurance coverage, could be counted on to provide a steady stream of funding to hospitals. The third-party payers brought in a lot of "new business" to hospitals. Hospitals responded with continued growth and expansion.

The availability of health insurance meant that by the middle of the twentieth century, more people were not only willing to go to the hospital but were prepared to stay there for days (before the surge of hospital-based infections caused doctors to discharge patients sooner). There was a broad consensus that the hospital sector needed to expand and add new beds.

In passing Medicare legislation, the government took steps to ensure that the funds would go to high-quality hospitals. It decreed that Medicare funds could only go to hospitals accredited by the Joint Commission. (Remember, this is the voluntary association created to upgrade standards.) This resulted in a degree of reorganization of the hospital sector. Hospitals that could not pass a review by the Joint Commission were forced to close. They could not compete with hospitals eager to emphasize they had received this stamp of approval in the literature they produced to describe themselves.

RISING COSTS OF CARE

Health policy analysts watched healthcare costs increase in response to the introduction of Medicare and Medicaid but didn't try to monitor costs until 1978. This was when the first piece of legislation aimed at cost control came into existence: the Healthcare Common Procedure Coding System (HCPCS). It introduced a two-level coding system to be used for reimbursement and data-collection purposes. Level I codes were to cover medical procedures in and out of the hospital; Level II codes were to cover products and supplies used in the care of patients in the hospital and other things, such as ambulance services and prosthetic devices. The Level I code is built on the Current Procedural Terminology (CPT) code developed by the AMA (discussed in the previous chapter).

The next piece of legislation aimed at controlling rising healthcare costs came in 1983 in an amendment to the Social Security Act that introduced a major change in Medicare reimbursement. This turned out to be significant not only because Medicare had a vast number of enrollees but because the other third-party payers, Medicaid, and private insurers were ready to adopt the Medicare reimbursement schedule.

In passing this legislation, policy analysts were responding to the determination that paying hospitals based on *charges* rather than *costs* was responsible for rising expenditures. This was when Medicare established a reimbursement schedule based on the diagnoses with which patients were admitted to the hospital. Amazingly, all possible diagnostic categories were subsumed into 467 Diagnostic Related Groups (DRGs), plus a few more catchall categories. (The current number is 767.) Medicare would now pay a set amount of money for all goods and services included under the DRG. If the hospital could do whatever was necessary for less than the DRG payment, it got to keep the extra funds. If the funds were insufficient, the hospital simply had to find a way to cover that.

Hospitals in communities with a high proportion of poor people complained that DRG reimbursement was insufficient to cover their costs because their patients invariably presented with more complications than those in middle-class communities. Health policymakers didn't dispute that, which led to the Disproportionate Share Hospital (DSH) adjustment, passed in 1985. There have been repeated efforts to discontinue these payments in response to legislation promising universal coverage. Since that has yet to happen, the DSH legislation keeps getting renewed.

Another intervention to deal with the needs of poor, uninsured patients designed to keep them out of the hospital came in the form of health centers supported by the Health Resources and Services Administration (HRSA), an agency established in 1982. Operating under the auspices of HHS, HRSA was authorized to provide funding through grants for which the health centers had to apply. A successful application resulted in being designated a Federally Qualified Health Center (FQHC). To qualify for funding, the centers were required to show that they were serving a medically underserved population. This could include migrant workers, homeless persons, or public-housing residents.

The legislation required that the centers be governed by a community board representing the population being served. They were required to use a sliding-scale fee system based on family size and income. Being designated an FQHC brought a variety of benefits. For a start, the HRSA drug-pricing program allowed the centers to qualify for a 25 to 50 percent discount on drugs and vaccines. The centers could serve as sites where National Health Service Corps (NHSC) medical, dental, and mental health providers could earn educational loan repayment benefits (up to $170,000) at no cost to the centers. Providers are also covered by federally supported malpractice insurance.

Evaluations revealed that the FQHCs were doing exactly what they were created to do. Does that mean that most observers are satisfied to see this happening? Not exactly. They agree that the FQHCs work well. It is just that there is no assurance that they are being established in all the places they are needed. Distribution is unsystematic because it is voluntary and depends on community initiative and capability. It varies for many reasons, including density, meaning there are no organized groups in the community to represent the residents' interests.

Centers that come into existence meeting the criteria for this designation but do not apply for it are known as "look-alike" centers. They qualify for some of the benefits but not all. Evidence shows that a growing number of hospitals are creating look-alike centers as independent, nonprofit organizations so they can outsource poor patients to them.[4]

The introduction of DRGs did not have the anticipated cost-reduction effect. That brought about the Combined Reconciliation Act of 1986, which instituted the annual re-evaluation of DRGs. The law also required hospitals to use the international disease classification system (IC-10-CM) and the associated coding system (ICD-10-PCS) by 2015. This was intended to make US mortality and morbidity statistics comparable to international statistics based on a system many other countries had already adopted. Hospital administrators complained that this requirement presented a huge financial burden. It is important to recognize that the legislation was passed at a time when computers were not nearly as well-developed and no software program existed. That, plus the need to train staff to use the new data-collection system, really did add up to a big expense. However, over the next few years, things settled down as consensus developed on which computers and software programs to use.

Hospital administrators were even more upset about another piece of legislation passed at the same time, the Emergency Medical Treatment and Labor Act (EMTALA), which prohibits hospitals from turning patients away from the emergency room before stabilizing them, even if they are unable to pay for their care. News media featured stories about uninsured patients admitted to the intensive care unit for extended periods, with the hospital having to pick up the bill.

The next and most significant piece of healthcare-oriented legislation since Medicare and Medicaid were passed was the 2010 Patient Protection and Affordable Care Act (ACA). The combined effect of the mandate that everyone in the country obtains health insurance produced an influx of new enrollees, even though it was overturned two years later. The expansion of Medicaid in many, but not all, states produced an even more substantial increase in hospital admissions.

The ACA had some other effects on the hospital sector. One was to prohibit new "specialty hospitals." There were about 200 in existence at the time. Community and public hospitals argued that specialty hospitals, which generally focus on a particular form of treatment, typically cardiac and orthopedic surgery, siphon off patients at lower risk of complications. Such hospitals provide high-quality care largely because they do not accept patients whose care promises to be complex and more expensive to treat, leaving those patients to be cared for by traditional community hospitals.

THE SHORTER LENGTH OF STAY

Going back to the initial effect of DRGs, hospitals came up with a number of ways to compensate for the financial losses they knew would come with the DRG reimbursement arrangement. One mechanism was the reduction in the number of days (*length of stay*) a person stayed in the hospital. In 1980, people stayed an average of 7.5 days; by 2010, they stayed for 4.8 days.[5] (The 2022 length of stay is 4.5 days.) Initially, the news media featured scary stories about hospitals discharging patients "quicker and sicker." A particularly sensational depiction featured by the news media was of a discharged patient sitting in a wheelchair in the hospital's driveway, waiting to be picked up and looking too sick to move. However, things change. As already noted, discharging patients as soon as possible became common practice, with everyone agreeing that doing so protects patients from acquiring a hospital-based infection and aids recovery by allowing patients the comfort of sleeping in their own beds and getting more rest.

The most innovative tactic hospitals came up with to make up for lost earnings was admitting patients for less than twenty-four hours. Since DRGs cover *inpatient* care but not *outpatient* care, hospitals could charge rates that were not so closely monitored for treating patients on an outpatient basis. They built new units inside hospitals for this purpose. They also began building freestanding outpatient clinics both near and far from the parent hospital.

The upshot was that the patients admitted to the hospital were now more seriously ill, requiring increased intensity of services, leading, in turn, to increased costs.

HOSPITALS AND QUALITY OF CARE

The quality of hospital care attracted a great deal of attention in response to the shocking assessment released by the Institute of Medicine (IOM) in 1999, reporting that errors in hospital care were responsible for an annual loss of 44,000 lives. Although some challenged that number, the report spurred academics, government agencies, and various nonprofit entities to act—to work on creating quality measures.

The Centers for Medicare and Medicaid Services (CMS) followed up in 2005 with the Hospital Compare initiative. This evaluation instrument was based on sixty-four indicators that led to a five-star rating system. By 2020, the number of indicators had grown to 150. Hospital representatives argued that the star rating system oversimplified complex treatment procedures. One of the most controversial indicators was readmission. The most advanced academic hospitals complained that the patients they treat are admitted with the most complicated conditions and, therefore, at greater risk of readmission. The Health Compare rating system meant these hospitals ended up with lower ratings, which translated into lower reimbursements. That did lead to some changes in the instrument, although government spokespersons were not ready to discard it because they believed it was producing positive results. According to the Secretary of Health and Human Services serving at that time,

> Every year, about 2.6 million seniors—or nearly one in five hospitalized Medicare enrollees—are readmitted within 30 days of discharge, at a cost of more than $26 billion to the Medicare program. Many of these readmissions stem from preventable problems.[6]

Another effort to address quality came from the Agency for Healthcare Research and Quality (AHRQ), which released a set of quality indicators in 2003 that it updated in 2008. Its website offers a consumer guide to hospital quality, which states that consumers can examine "hundreds of measures" that focus on the quality of inpatient care. It goes on to say that the list has multiple indicators: (1) patient safety, (2) effectiveness, (3) patient-centeredness, (4) timeliness, (5) efficiency, and (6) equity. Physicians are required to produce the information used to construct these domains in response to a range of different data-collection instruments. Needless to say, physicians and hospitals see this as an administrative burden.

The question is: To what extent do prospective patients rely on government sources for information on hospital quality? Critics of "consumer-driven" health care continue to argue that patients are not qualified to take on this task—no matter how much information anyone, whether it's government agencies or private sector entities, is ready to provide. The US News and World Report evaluation of hospitals introduced in 1990 may be the most familiar private-sector source. While it is unclear how many prospective patients refer to it, hospital administrators and doctors regularly debunk its ratings but are ready to use them in advertising when they are favorable. This is in recognition of the fact that the public is far more inclined to rely on such sources than search less user-friendly government sources.

We will get back to the idea that patients can be convinced to shop for less expensive health care at the end of this chapter. For now, I will note that Americans have lost trust in most social institutions, including government agencies. They are readier to turn to their physicians, friends, and relatives for advice rather than "experts" of any stripe. (See Marioua and Bozic for a history of the quality movement.[7])

GROWTH OF THE FOR-PROFIT HOSPITAL SECTOR

Let us now turn back to the third basic distinguishing hospital characteristic mentioned at the beginning of this chapter: hospital ownership. Government statistics continue to differentiate between nonprofit and for-profit community hospitals. The Federation of American Hospitals (FAH), established in 1966 to represent for-profit hospitals, makes clear that the interests of its member hospitals are not identical to those of hospitals and hospital systems belonging to the American Hospital Association (AHA). The FAH states that it represents "investor-owned hospitals" in contrast to "nonprofit hospitals" associated with the AHA. The FAH further asserts that it represents "tax-paying community hospitals and health systems."

FAH representatives maintain that what they do is socially beneficial because the performance of investor-owned hospitals pressures nonprofit hospitals to be more efficient. This, they say, serves to bring down prices. Critics counter by arguing that investor-owned hospital corporations employ tactics that nonprofit hospitals are not prepared to adopt and that the tactics deserve greater scrutiny. This includes the fact that investor-owned hospitals are far more likely to be established in suburban communities rather than the inner city, allowing them to treat healthier, wealthier patients. They typically do not have emergency rooms. They do little or no research and no medical education. They have lower patient-staff ratios, meaning they have lower personnel costs, which they achieve by employing fewer nurses with advanced training. Instead, they employ less-expensive, easily replaced "technicians" to do specific tasks such as taking blood pressure or giving "shots"—an approach grounded in a factory model of efficiency.

As an aside, when one highly respected university teaching hospital in an urban area with which I'm familiar tried this, it found that bringing in unskilled personnel who needed to be trained to carry out specific tasks increased the risk of mistakes—medication errors, inability to recognize indicators that something is not right, carelessness about the disposal of infectious materials, and so on. Yes, it had to do with who they hired. Some, certainly not all, of the new employees were burdened by the problems related to poverty in their communities, problems they brought with them to the job. They spent more time being dragged down by life's problems, sleeping on the job, for example, than concentrating on the work they were hired to do.

The drive for greater efficiency celebrated by the investor-owned hospital sector led to consolidation, meaning small hospitals, both for-profit and nonprofit, were absorbed by large corporate hospital networks. The primary benefit of consolidation is that it allows the networks to negotiate prices from a position of greater market power, reducing operating costs. There is no evidence to indicate that consolidation has led to lower prices. In fact, there is a large body of evidence indicating that it resulted in increased prices.[8]

Consolidation of hospitals in the for-profit sector received the most attention during the closing years of the twentieth century and early twenty-first century, revealing that, in some cases, consolidation had led to massive fraud. In June 2003, the US Department of Justice settled a suit with the Hospital Corporation of America (HCA) when it pled guilty to fourteen felonies and agreed to pay $1.7 billion in fines. The Justice Department alleged "that HCA systematically defrauded Medicare, Medicaid, and other federally funded healthcare programs through schemes dating back to the late 1980s."[9] It was the largest healthcare fraud case to date. The HCA, founded in 1968, was operating 343 hospitals, 136 outpatient surgery centers, and approximately 550 home-health sites by 1997. The CEO at the time was Rick Scott, formerly the governor of and now a Republican senator representing Florida.

A few years later, in 2006, the Tenet Healthcare Corporation, the second largest hospital chain, agreed to settle a Justice Department suit alleging unlawful billing practices for $900 million.[10] The scandal continued as investigative reporting found that doctors at one of the Tenet hospitals in California were performing unnecessary surgeries putting patients at risk for no medical reason.

Critics said that no one should be surprised to find hospitals operated on a for-profit basis engaged in such practices. (For a graphic account, see Marcia Mahar's *Money-Driven Medicine*.[11])

The HCA finds itself in the news once again in 2022, battling charges of fraud. The Service Employees International Union (SEIU) presented an investigative report to a representative in Congress alleging that the HCA overcharged Medicare at least $1.8 billion through excessive admissions. A whistle-blower's account reinforced the charge—a physician associated with a 400-bed HCA hospital in Miami said he was told he would lose his job if he did not admit more patients coming to the hospital's ER.[12]

Large hospital systems, with HCA and Tenet getting a special mention, reported huge profits in 2021. It turns out the profits were attributable in large part to "bailout" funding provided by the federal government to address the financial stress organizations experienced as a result of Covid-19. At the same time, some smaller hospitals failed because the bailout funds they received were not enough to cover their losses. Rural hospitals were especially hard hit.

The failure of rural hospitals is a problem that goes beyond concerns related to health care because hospitals in rural communities are major employers. When they fail, the economy in the area is affected because so many people lose their jobs, which has a spiraling effect, leading to business closers and a decline in population as people move away to seek employment.[13]

A growing concern revolves around private equity investment in hospital systems because, as noted in the previous chapter, the investors bring no healthcare experience.[14] This is an increasing trend since investors consider hospital systems to be a secure asset because hospital systems are recession resistant and projected to become more profitable due to increased demand as the population ages.

CONSOLIDATION OF NONPROFIT HOSPITALS

During the last couple of decades of the twentieth century, while the for-profit hospital scandals were unfolding, nonprofit hospitals were generally widely lauded for their contribution to the health of members of their communities. At the same time, business community members criticized them for being inefficient, pressing them to employ business practices. The nonprofit hospital sector took notice. Nonprofit hospitals did begin to act more like the for-profits. Large, established nonprofit hospitals started buying up smaller hospitals and forming networks. That gave them leverage to negotiate with suppliers and health insurance companies, just as investor-owned hospital networks were doing.

Responding to criticism of nonprofit hospitals' tax-exempt status, the ACA introduced a new set of rules aimed at tightening the requirements for claiming nonprofit status. The Social Security Administration recognizes 501(c)(3) nonprofit organizational status made by any organization that applies without requiring the organization to offer proof that it is not profiting from its activities. The fact that the ACA introduced rules to ensure that nonprofit hospitals actually fulfilled their commitment came as an unwelcome surprise. Nonprofit hospitals found that they were now required to have four clearly outlined policies in place and to make those policies public: (1) a community needs assessment to be conducted every three years; (2) a financial assistance policy; (3) limitation on charges; and (4) limitation on billing and collections. The community needs assessment policy was the most challenging. It meant hospitals would have to study the health needs in their community and work with community residents to develop a plan to address those needs. And they would have to show how they planned to provide evidence that they were, in fact, addressing those needs.

That hasn't worked out exactly as planned. According to some health policy analysts, nonprofit hospitals have been ready to meet "the letter of the law but not the spirit." Questions about the legitimacy of their nonprofit status have not stopped. One estimate of how much nonprofit hospitals spend on charity care indicates that they spend $2.30—less than the $3.80 for every $100 spent by for-profit hospitals. The researchers say a revised set of standards is needed.[15] Another group of researchers found that charity care represented 1.4 percent or less of operating expenses at half of all hospitals in 2020.[16]

The fact that nonprofit hospitals no longer enjoy the positive image they had in the past is confirmed by news media reports. The media has turned from reporting fraud perpetrated by investor-owned hospital chains to reporting on nonprofit hospital chains "hounding" patients to pay for the care they were entitled to get for free. An example comes in a 2022 *New York Times* story on the tactics used by Providence, one of the largest nonprofit hospital chains in the country. (The story also comes in the form of a podcast if you're interested.[17]) It seems that Providence's chief financial officer adopted the "Rev-up program" (short for "revenue up"), which came with a "detailed playbook for wringing money out of patients—even those who were supposed to receive free care." The staff was instructed to do the following: "'Ask every patient, every time,'. . . . Instead of using 'weak' phrases—like 'Would you mind paying?'—employees were told to ask how patients wanted to pay. Soliciting money 'is part of your role. It's not an option.'"[18]

Health insurance companies complain that networked hospitals, both for-profit and nonprofit, have grown so large that they now have an unfair negotiating advantage. They have said as far back as the early 2000s that there is no difference between for-profit and nonprofit hospitals and that both were making huge profits, with the only difference being that the nonprofits are tax-exempt. A study conducted by National Nurses United (NNU) reflects on this observation. It found that "Overall, the 100 most expensive U.S. hospitals charge from $1,120 to $1,808 for every $100 of their costs. Nationally, U.S. hospitals average $417 for every $100 of their costs, a markup that more than doubled over the past 20 years."[19]

THE CHARGEMASTER

Representatives of nonprofit as well as investor-owned hospitals continue to argue that they must find ways to cover the cost of caring for patients who cannot pay. The traditional way this was done was by writing it off as "bad debt," which Medicare reimburses at 65 percent. Hospital representatives claim that their debt burden is too great and that the 65 percent rebate is insufficient to cover their losses. That brings up the question of how they calculate those losses.

The prices hospitals charge when there is no negotiated third-party contract are based on a "chargemaster." This is the price list for all the goods and services they offer. The list can run to thousands of items. Each hospital comes up with a price for each of the items on the list. The lists are not comparable from one hospital to another. For example, one hospital can charge an outsized amount for gauze or toothpaste, and another can charge a similarly outsized amount for something else, aiming to cover other costs. And until recently, hospitals were not required to make their chargemasters public—to anyone. California was the only state to require it until 2021, when all hospitals, by law, were required to make their chargemaster prices public. This was done in response to calls for transparency to permit consumers to shop for hospital care based on price.

How well do you think that worked out? Critics said no one should have been surprised that the public couldn't figure out the codes used by hospitals for most items on their lists. And, as many health policy experts were quick to add, patients couldn't predict what goods and services they would require once they were hospitalized.

DIFFERENCES BY HOSPITAL OWNERSHIP

Although there is clear evidence that the differences between investor-owned and nonprofit hospitals are ebbing away, they may not be disappearing entirely. The picture is summed up by one group of researchers as follows:

> Nonprofit, for-profit, and government hospitals are all more likely to offer services when they are relatively profitable than when they are relatively unprofitable. However, for-profit hospitals are considerably more likely than others to provide services based on profitability. After hospital and market characteristics are adjusted for, nonprofit hospitals offer relatively unprofitable services more than for-profit hospitals and less than government hospitals. Profitable services typically exhibit the opposite pattern. For-profit hospitals are also more likely to adopt or discontinue services consistent with changes in service profitability

than are nonprofits, which in turn are more likely to do so than government hospitals.[20]

Researchers studying the development of for-profit hospitals across four nations offer a noteworthy assessment comparing the performance of for-profit versus nonprofit hospitals in the title of their article: "For-Profit Hospitals Have Thrived Because of Generous Public Reimbursement Schemes, Not Greater Efficiency: A Multi-Country Case Study."[21]

Then there are research findings comparing the care offered by private hospitals versus government-operated hospitals. A study reporting on veterans admitted to a VA hospital states that patients taken to a VA hospital are

> 46 percent less likely to die within 28 days of the ambulance ride than veterans who are taken to a private hospital, new research shows. Care in a V.A. hospitals also costs 21 percent less than those first 28 days, and the cumulative differential endures over time. . . . A possible explanation is that private hospitals, which charge fees for services, 'may be motivated to provide care that is highly reimbursed and avoid care that is not.[22]

While the three pieces of research I've just referenced are not enough to revise understandings about hospital ownership, they are thought-provoking and deserving of further consideration because they respond to some long-standing dogmas. Government-run organizations are constantly criticized for being far less efficient than organizations operated by the private sector. And investor-owned organizations are regularly touted as being more efficient than nonprofit organizations.

OTHER HEALTHCARE ORGANIZATIONS

One of the basic differentiating characteristics used in discussing healthcare facilities, *length of stay,* depends on whether the patients are *ambulatory* (able to walk) and expected to be there for a short stay or *bedridden* and expected to be there for an extended stay. Nursing homes, which are considered long-term stay facilities, have come under scrutiny because they have been growing in number in response to rising numbers of people who cannot care for themselves. In addition to the increasing number of people who need nursing home care because of problems associated with aging, there is the devastation that chronic illness in younger populations causes, for example, developmental disabilities, paralysis due to spinal injury, psychiatric problems, and so forth. The fact that modern medicine can perform miracles in saving people who would not have survived years ago does not necessarily mean that those who are saved can lead normal, healthy lives and live independently. Many require twenty-four-hour care and/or care lasting years.

Medicare helps pay for care in a long-stay facility but only after a patient is discharged from the hospital. There was considerable interest in the performance of nursing homes a few decades ago. The homes owned by for-profit chains were consistently found to have more violations than nonprofit or government-owned nursing homes. It is unclear whether this continues to be the case because the question has not been addressed in recent years.

The Covid-19 epidemic was especially hard on nursing home residents. Their mortality rate was far higher than it was for any other identifiable demographic category. This has returned focus on nursing home care, causing politicians to call for increased oversight. Years of academic research and investigative reporting indicating that the patient-staff ratio is inadequate in many nursing homes has finally attracted the attention of lawmakers, largely in response to the impact of Covid. As a first step, Congress requested a Government Accountability Office (GAO) probe of nursing homes.

· Home health care has been supported and, in fact, promoted, albeit with some trepidation, by health policymakers as a good alternative to residential nursing home care. Home health care is much less expensive than nursing home care because people stay in their own homes, and health workers go in for a few hours at a time. Also, virtually everyone prefers to stay in their own home. The fear is that too many people will opt for this form of care. In the past, wives, daughters, and other female relatives provided such care out of a sense of duty. Given that women have careers and are less willing to do this kind of work or cannot afford to do it because they need to earn a living means that policymakers continue to be concerned that the government will have to do something about the situation.

Medicare pays for hospice care when the doctor asserts that the patient has six months or less to live. Curative care is no longer provided. Hospice care has been expanding and has changed over the years. A ProPublica report tells us the first hospice opened in the United States in 1974.[23] It says this sector "has evolved from a constellation of charities, mostly reliant on volunteers, into a $22 billion juggernaut funded almost entirely by taxpayers." The report states that the number of hospice organizations owned by private-equity firms tripled between 2011 and 2019. The report is an exposé that goes on to reveal all kinds of malfeasance: bribes to doctors, overdosed patients, Medicare fraud, and pressure on employees to sign up people who don't qualify for hospice care, to name a few practices. It also documents the failure of the courts to hold the fraudsters accountable. A disheartened lawyer for whistle-blowers is quoted offering a shrewd assessment of the situation—as a "system with a capitalist payee and a socialist payer."

While you probably think you wouldn't want to hear about end-of-life care in any detail, I assure you the ProPublica report makes for an engrossing, if disenchanting, read—more like a manuscript that would make a great movie script about a colossal scam.

As if you haven't had enough bad news about private sector investors, it appears that yet one more category of healthcare system participants to be investigated and charged with overcharging are ambulance companies. Researchers who compared the billing practices of private- and public-sector ambulances found that 28 percent of transports by private-sector companies resulted in surprise bills.[24] Unfortunately, the new No Surprises Act of 2022 does not apply to ambulance services.

INITIATIVES AIMED AT REDUCING COSTS

Policies aimed at increasing quality and reducing hospital costs continue to be explored. The Center for American Progress identifies six policies that seem to cover most of the bases aimed at lowering the cost of hospital care: (1) ending abusive hospital billing practices, the most egregious being *surprise billing* (which, as just mentioned, was addressed by a bill legislated in 2022); (2) reference pricing. This policy is intended to encourage patients to use lower-cost providers to pressure other providers to lower their prices; (3) rate regulation. Maryland is the only state in the country that has adopted an "all-payer" reimbursement system that pays all third-party payers at the Medicare rate; (4) price transparency. This is intended to be used by insurers and employers to direct patients to lower-cost providers; (5) more anti-trust enforcement; and (6) site-neutral payment. This would mean reimbursement would be the same regardless of whether the procedure took place in an inpatient or outpatient facility.[25]

Much of the advice depends on the willingness of prospective patients to act as "consumers." What this suggests to me is that if prospective patients have not been ready to embrace the consumer role despite repeated efforts to convince them to do so, and the fact that promises of increased efficiency based on greater reliance on business practices have not brought lower prices, we need to turn to other solutions that I suggest you wait to consider until you finish reading the last chapter.

In the meantime, for an irreverent take on healthcare system billing and instructions consumers can employ to fight off surprise charges, check out Dan Weissmann's Kaiser Health News podcast, "Can They Freaking Do That?!?"[26]

Chapter 7

Pharmaceuticals

As I said when we began this discussion, people in this country disagree about a lot of things these days, so it's interesting to see so much agreement about the pharmaceutical industry. A 2019 Gallup poll found it to be the "most poorly regarded industry in Americans' eyes, ranking it last on a list of 25 industries."[1] The federal government came in second to last, and the healthcare industry came in third to last. My shorthand interpretation, for now, is that this has something to do with something to which I have alluded a couple of times already, namely, that Americans have lost confidence in the country's social institutions. And as I said, this has serious consequences, including consequences for health, something we will get back to in the final chapter.

Consistent with that observation, I'll add a slight correction to the idea that so many of us agree about the pharmaceutical industry. About 80 percent of us agree that the cost of drugs is unreasonable.[2] There's a fair amount of consensus on why the cost is so high—68 percent of Americans say it is due to research and development costs, and 52 percent say it is due to marketing and advertising. It's when people are asked who is best qualified to fix the problem that consensus falls apart and Americans go to their political corners to point fingers and make accusations.

The introduction of the Covid vaccine illustrates what disagreements in this country look like these days. Many people celebrated the Pfizer and Moderna vaccines based on mRNA (*messenger ribonucleic acid*) as a profound scientific breakthrough. There were also those who reacted by claiming it would cause infertility or alter one's DNA. Although there was no evidence for that, those claims sounded like they could have a grain of rationality behind them. Then there were the far more creative allegations, for example, that the vaccines carried microchips to allow the elite to control humanity, or that the vaccines were intended to create a Civil Registry, allowing the government to control society, or that Bill Gates was behind it so that he could surveil the population.

It's a lot easier and more entertaining to indulge in conspiracy theories than it is to do the work required to understand the data confirming the vaccine's value. And it takes some effort to work out why the price of drugs is so high in this country, higher than anywhere else in the world. That's exactly what we'll try to do next, tracking where the money comes from and who it goes to as drugs are developed, manufactured, distributed, and finally sold.

STEPS INVOLVED IN CREATING A DRUG

In taking a closer look at the process drugs go through before they appear in the pharmacy ready for us to take home, let's begin by identifying who is involved at each step. It begins with the *discovery stage*, which starts with researchers affiliated with academic institutions designing lab research projects with the expectation of finding a molecular reaction with the potential of a health benefit. Most apply for National Institutes of Health (NIH) funding to support this work. If they come up with promising results, they move on to test their findings on lab animals. This is the *pre-clinical* stage. In short, the preliminary research leading to findings that may ultimately result in a drug is generally funded by the public sector.

Publishing findings or otherwise sharing lab research results with colleagues attracts the attention of pharmaceutical companies interested in translating those results into marketable products. Researchers in university settings are not set up to manufacture and sell drugs. They expect to hand over their discovery to a major corporation with the resources to turn their research results into an actual drug.

Academic researchers may seek a patent for the chemical composition of their discovery as individuals or in partnership with their university. Assuming a pharmaceutical company expresses interest, the researchers may negotiate compensation to transfer ownership of the patent. Or they may allow the pharmaceutical company to obtain patents for their research findings without expecting any financial reward. In any case, the discovery generally becomes privately owned, and whatever monetary gains come from the discovery go to the patent holders.

The initial patent application is to the US Patent and Trademark Office (PTO), which issues three kinds of patents: utility, design, and plant (yes, things that grow in the ground). Most patent seekers apply for the utility patent, which confers intellectual property protection. The PTO charges a series of fees, starting with an application fee, which varies depending on the size of the organization making the application, lawyers' fees, and maintenance fees, with the first renewal after three and one-half years. Additional renewal fees are required after this initial period; this runs into thousands of dollars.

Once a pharmaceutical company becomes involved, the drug development process enters the *clinical stage*, which involves testing—what is now considered a new drug—on human beings. Clinical testing has three basic phases plus a fourth phase that may or may not be completed. During phase one, the focus is on *safety* and involves, on average, about thirty healthy volunteers. The purpose is to determine the appropriate dose, how it should be administered, and basic information on the body's reaction to the treatment. Phase two is about *efficacy*. It typically involves around 500 patients who have a particular illness. This phase is meant to study the treatment's effects and determine whether it offers any benefit. If it is found to do so, the clinical trial moves on to the third phase, the *clinical benefit* phase, which typically involves about 5,000 patients. The purpose is to compare the newly identified treatment with existing treatments. The trials are double-blinded, meaning that neither the patients nor the doctors doing the evaluations know which patients are getting the treatment and which are getting a placebo. The fourth phase comes after the drug is approved. Drug companies are expected to gather more information on safety and efficacy, something they may or may not do.

The *clinical benefit* testing phase is expensive because it involves so many people and takes years to complete, more or less time depending on how long it takes for the effects of the treatments to manifest themselves. Pharmaceutical companies are not expected to report the costs of conducting clinical trials. But cost has become an issue, with some observers arguing that it has become prohibitive. One widely cited study puts the average cost at $19 million per clinical study.[3] The researchers who reported this sum examined 225 studies to determine costs. They found huge differences in costs depending on two variables: the number of patients, which varied from two to 8,442; and the number of clinic visits the research subjects were required to make, which was between two to 166.

The cost of carrying out expensive clinical studies has not discouraged interested parties. The number of trials continues to increase. The NIH, which keeps track of the number of clinical trials, listed 435,727 trials in fifty states and 221 countries as of March 2021; 177,111 were drug trials.[4] The other trials involved behavioral interventions, surgical procedures, and devices.

Pharmaceutical companies do not always conduct their own clinical trials. Currently, about two-thirds are outsourced. Privately owned clinical trial organizations do the recruiting of patients, work to retain the patients they recruit, and ultimately conduct the trials. As you might expect, the fact that pharmaceutical companies are not directly involved raises concerns about quality and oversight. Private-sector clinical trial work is lucrative but not something that is being tracked.

As an aside, would you be surprised to find that private equity firms are getting into this business?[5] As you are already aware, we keep hearing about the extent to which ownership of healthcare sector entities is moving in this direction and the rising level of concern this is causing.

Assuming the clinical trials indicate that the drug being tested shows evidence of benefiting patients and has no serious negative side effects, the pharmaceutical company applies to the Federal Drug Administration (FDA) for a patent. In many instances, this happens much earlier in the process to prevent other companies from trying to develop the drug. The FDA patent establishes exclusivity, which the US Patent and Trademark Office patent does not cover. The FDA patent gives the holder the exclusive right to make and sell the product for approximately twenty years. The FDA lists all approved pharmaceutical products in something called the Orange Book.

Criticism of the patenting system abounds. The fundamental objection is that the exclusivity benefit creates government-sanctioned monopolies.

"The original purpose of the patent system was to encourage and incentivize innovation. Most companies are no longer innovating new medications but monopolizing existing ones. It is estimated that between 78% and 80% of new patent applications are not for new medicines."[6]

More objectionable, in the view of some, is the fact that patents are being extended for an unreasonable amount of time and for questionable reasons. For example, an analysis of the ten best-selling drugs in 2019 found that, on average, the drugs were covered by more than sixty-nine patents with 37.5 years of patent protection. A few companies have come in for particular reproach. For example, AbbVie has come under fire for exploiting the patent system for Humira, filing over 250 patents costing the country $19 billion because success in obtaining all those patent applications prevents generic and biosimilar competition. The company also filed over 150 patents for Imbruvica, costing the health system $41 billion. Teva, another major pharmaceutical company, is charged with *product hopping*, meaning it switched patents to a version of the drug that is the same but with a change in dosage. That produced a two-and-a-half-year delay and resulted in between $4.3 billion and $6.5 billion in excess costs to the health system.

How the FDA is funded has been attracting increased criticism of late. Before 1992, the FDA was publicly funded. Since then, it has relied on *user fees* paid by pharmaceutical companies whose patent applications the FDA evaluates. The *New York Times* reports that "The pharmaceutical industry finances about 75% of the agency's drug division."[7] That, in turn, has led some observers to note that the amount of money involved is propelling the "revolving door" between the FDA and pharmaceutical industry as high-level administrators leave the FDA for lucrative jobs with drug companies, bringing connections and knowledge of how the FDA operates with them.

Generic Drugs

The Hatch-Waxman Act of 1984 was legislated to speed up the approval of generic drugs in an effort to eliminate the hold pharmaceutical companies have on brand-name drug prices due to patents. Before the law was passed, 20 percent of drugs were generic; as of 2021, 89 percent are.[8]

Pharmaceutical companies responded to the Hatch-Waxman Act by applying for additional patents to extend the time they are in a position to prevent companies that make generic versions of the patented drug from producing it. They also came up with various ethically questionable approaches for accomplishing this. One is *pay-for-delay*. This is when a brand-name drug company pays a generic company to hold off on producing the generic. The Federal Trade Commission (FTC) estimates this costs the country $3.5 billion in higher drug costs per year.

Another method relies on *citizen petitions* meant to allow ordinary citizens to ask the FDA to delay action on pending generic drug applications. The citizens in 92 percent of the cases have turned out to be corporations. The brand-name pharmaceutical companies file the petitions close to the patent expiration date, thus gaining another 150 days of exclusivity.

A third method is to apply for an *authorized generic* patent. This is when the company selling the brand-name drug turns it into a generic. Applying for this patent gives the brand-name company 180 days of exclusivity, barring other companies from producing it.

Pharmaceutical companies may also restrict access to samples that generic companies need to conduct bioequivalent testing. The brand-name companies cite the FDA requirement preventing patients who will not benefit from the drug from buying it. This is called the Risk Evaluation and Mitigation Strategies program. But brand-name companies use it to keep generic companies from studying the components in the drug they are interested in producing, thus preventing it from coming to market.

The FDA estimates that generics saved the country about $293 million in 2018; other estimates indicate that the savings were nearly $2 trillion over the preceding decade.[9] The entry of additional generic companies meant that competition caused prices to fall 37 percent between 2014 and 2018, while branded drug prices increased more than 60 percent.

Orphan Drugs

The Orphan Drug Act of 1983 was passed to incentivize pharmaceutical companies to develop drugs to treat illnesses affecting small numbers of people in the country, numbering 200,000 or fewer. The FDA grants seven years of exclusivity and manages a program that awards a 50 percent tax credit. Drug companies have applied for and received orphan designations for 5,099 drugs and biologics between 1983 and 2019.[10]

PHARMACY BENEFIT MANAGERS

Pharmaceutical companies do not deal directly with persons who consume their products and don't even deal with the pharmacies that sell those products. They rely on wholesalers known as pharmacy benefit managers (PBMs). PBMs handle about 92 percent of the drugs distributed in the United States.[11]

PBMs purchase brand-name drugs from pharmaceutical companies at a negotiated discount, which is kept confidential, and sell the drugs to pharmacies at a higher price. They keep this difference as profit. However, handling branded drugs is not their primary source of profit. They are more active in the generic drug market and derive more significant profit because generics now comprise 90 percent of retail prescription purchases. The end result is that for every $100 spent at the pharmacy, $41 goes to the intermediary in the supply chain.

The PBMs have been found to engage in practices that have come under scrutiny. One is *spread pricing*, which involves paying the pharmacy one price and charging the health insurance company a higher price. Another technique is the *clawback*, which means PBMs are charging pharmacies additional fees for doing business with them.

Congress has taken notice of the role PBMs play and how much it costs the government. A study comparing what Medicare paid for prescriptions filled at a Costco pharmacy and plans administered through PBMs indicates that Medicare overpaid by 43 percent to the PBMs.[12]

Congress is considering various reforms. One would prevent PBMs and health insurance plans from collecting rebates from drug makers. Another involves requiring the FTC to look into anti-competitive behavior resulting from the consolidation of the PBM industry. Over the last decade, three companies have come to control 80 percent of the market, two of which are also major health insurance companies; this includes Caremark (CVS Health), Express Scripts (Cigna), and OptumRx (UnitedHealth).

GETTING DRUGS TO MARKET SOONER

Accelerated approval of new drugs was established in 1992 in response to the AIDS crisis. It proved very effective. The same approval process was invoked when Covid vaccines came into existence. However, some observers have begun to question the need for accelerated approval in non-public health emergencies. Some observers blame user fees collected by the FDA for the agency's willingness to grant accelerated approval without better evidence. It is becoming a far more common path, with fourteen out of fifty approvals in 2021 compared with four out of fifty-nine in 2018. Critics claim that this is due to having a pharma-funded FDA.[13]

The approval of the Alzheimer's drug Aduhelm is currently at the center of this debate. Medicare won't pay for it, and doctors at many prestigious hospitals won't offer it. They argue that it is only marginally effective and its price, $28,200 for a year's course of treatment, is unacceptable. The matter may move to court to be settled.

PHARMACIES

That brings us to the final set of participants in the drug distribution system, pharmacies. Pharmacies have been consolidating into pharmacy chains. The top seven account for nearly 70 percent of dispensing revenue from a total of $501 billion.[14]

The business practices the pharmacy industry engages in have come under scrutiny. This includes illegal importation of drugs from developing countries, promoting drugs off-label, false billing, and drug switching. But these practices aren't attracting as much attention as the practices major pharmaceutical companies engage in.

PHARMACEUTICAL COMPANIES AND THE COVID-19 VACCINE

The fact that the Covid vaccine was developed through a government-pharmaceutical industry partnership has been lauded as an effective mechanism for addressing a national crisis. Moderna, Sanofi, Novavax, and Johnson & Johnson got billions of dollars to develop the vaccine. Pfizer did not accept funds from the US government but did receive $445 million from the German government. At the same time, Pfizer spent $25 million "in lobbying and payments to 19 lobbying firms, pushing for legislation to protect its products and promote more robust U.S. vaccination programs."[15] It could afford this expenditure given that it recorded a $7.8 billion profit for its vaccine in 2021. Furthermore, the US government agreed to buy 1.6 billion additional doses over the next year.

Pfizer had abandoned the vaccine business because it did not produce enough profit. But it got into the business again when it purchased Wyeth, which made a highly profitable vaccine against pneumonia and ear infections.

Pfizer is now a "global powerhouse" and moving toward seeking licensure for drugs to treat a variety of diseases and infections.

Pfizer's success may be partially responsible for increased interest in the Bayh–Dole Act of 1980, which gave federal agencies *march-in* rights.[16] The law, which has never been invoked, gives government agencies the right to take patent licensure for themselves. The argument behind this movement is that the NIH scientists invented a key feature of Pfizer's vaccine. This threat may help explain the amount of money and effort Pfizer has devoted to lobbying.

The success of the government-pharmaceutical sector partnership in bringing the Covid vaccine into existence has also prompted some legislators to sponsor something called the Pasteur Act, which carries a $6 billion price tag. The idea is that the government would give pharmaceutical companies up-front payment in exchange for unlimited access to new, FDA-approved antibiotics. This is being considered because drug companies have stopped doing research to identify new antibiotics. Meanwhile, older, less-effective antibiotics are being overused, resulting in antibiotic resistance. While many observers, including politicians and doctors, think the up-front payment idea is laudable, there is also some opposition. Critics say the problem is the *noninferiority* tenet, which allows the FDA to approve drugs that are less effective than existing ones. They argue that this would be a giveaway to pharmaceutical companies since they would not have to prove the efficacy of the new drugs they present for approval. Others take the position that requiring clinical trials in this instance is unacceptable because clinical trial procedures would require giving placebos to persons suffering from an antibiotic-resistant infection, which they say is unconscionable.

I'll let you determine where you stand with regard to these arguments.

WHY DRUGS ARE SO EXPENSIVE

This may be a good place to stop to review the factors that account for the high cost of drugs. The cost of development of drugs is estimated to be around $3 billion per new drug by some accounts. One of the major reasons to explain why pharmaceutical companies charge so much for the drugs they sell is the high failure rate. Only 10 to 20 percent of all drugs tested come to market. Then there is the length of time it takes from the pre-clinical testing stage to final approval, which is, on average, about twelve years, during which the company is spending money on testing but is not making money on the product. Given this reality, the unfortunate result, according to some knowledgeable observers, is that "the costs of development are inversely proportional to the incremental benefit provided by the new drug, since it takes trials with larger sample size, and greater number of trials to secure regulatory approval."[17]

The high cost of bringing a drug to market, combined with the fact that prescription drugs are essential, means that pharmaceutical companies are spending money lobbying to safeguard their existence and profitability. In 2018, they spent approximately $220 billion lobbying Congress. It is worth mentioning that pharmaceutical companies are global, meaning they produce their products in various countries, so the production process is difficult to monitor. The fact that they are global makes it difficult to establish control over pricing.

Pharmaceutical companies are also spending a fortune on advertising. Only one other country besides the United States permits direct-to-consumer advertising: New Zealand. You may or may not have noticed the similarity in the scripts you hear. They all say one should consult with one's doctor about the drug. That is in response to how the law is written to permit advertising. The result, according to doctors, is they must spend too much time explaining why a particular drug is not appropriate to the patient's condition, but patients are convinced they need it. Doctors say such conversations don't always turn out well, and patients leave feeling deprived and distrustful.

According to some observers, Congress has not pushed back, at least not nearly enough, to prevent brand-name pharmaceutical companies from monopolizing the production and sale of particular drugs over extended periods. And it has done little to restrict pharmaceutical industry mergers. Researchers say mergers constitute a growing concern because merged companies spend less on research and quell competition by buying out innovative peers and smaller start-ups.[18]

You might imagine that the negative attention major drug companies are receiving would cause them to be more careful about attracting even more criticism, but they just seem to come up with more schemes, some more difficult to curb than others. For example, one recently identified scheme involves pharmaceutical companies contributing to patient-assistance charities but earmarking the donations for treating a particular condition, one that employs the drug they produce. This avoids the anti-kick-back statute prohibiting companies from offering to cover Medicare enrollees' out-of-pocket costs for drugs they produce.

Unethical and illegal behavior is widespread, with 85 percent of pharmaceutical companies being penalized for fraud. Pharmaceutical companies paid $33 billion in fines between January 2003 and December 2016. GlaxoSmithKline paid nearly $10 billion. Pfizer paid $3 billion, and Johnson and Johnson paid $2.7 billion. The co-author of the study tracking the fines makes the following observation:

The pharmaceutical industry is unique in that all large pharmaceutical firms explicitly state that they are focused on promoting patient welfare, yet the majority of large pharmaceutical firms engage in illegal activities that harm patient welfare.[19]

WHERE THINGS STAND IN TRYING
TO CONTROL COSTS

The Inflation Reduction Act of 2022, which turns out to be the most significant piece of health legislation since the passage of the Affordable Care Act (ACA), includes a list of provisions directed at the pharmaceutical sector. It focuses on drugs used by people on Medicare, capping out-of-pocket spending on Part D to $2,000. It also requires drug companies to pay rebates to Medicare if prices rise faster than inflation for drugs; it caps the cost of insulin at $35; it eliminates cost-sharing for adult vaccines; and it expands eligibility for full benefits under the Part D Low-Income Subsidy Program.

The most significant change, however, is the requirement that the Secretary of the Department of Health and Human Services (HHS) negotiate the price of brand-name drugs, but not generics or biosimilars, covered under Medicare Part D as of 2026 and Medicare Part B as of 2028. This is to occur in stages, with negotiations over ten drugs in 2026; fifteen drugs in 2027; fifteen in Part D, and twenty in Part B in 2029. The drugs are to be selected from a list of those with the highest Medicare Part D spending. This legislation overrides the nearly six-decade prohibition in the original Medicare legislation preventing Medicare from negotiating over drug prices.

Other approaches considered by Congress that have come and gone include *international reference pricing*, that is, setting prices for drugs in the United States based on what other countries pay. Legal challenges stood in the way in that case. Another approach still being considered involves addressing the gap between the *list price* and the *net price* with the aim of reducing the price to consumers, not to the health insurance companies.

Finally, there is the approach that depends on adopting the negotiating arrangements used by other government health plans. The Government Accountability Office (GAO) conducted a review, in 2017, of the prices the US Department of Veterans Affairs (VA) paid for 399 drugs compared to what participants in Medicare Part D plans paid. The VA paid 75 percent less for 106 brand-name drugs and 50 percent less for another set of 233 brand-name drugs. It paid 68 percent less for generic drugs. The GAO did not take a stand on adopting the VA's price list, but it did make a critical observation, namely, that the VA buys directly from the manufacturers, bypassing the intermediaries. It's unclear why legislators haven't been more interested in adopting the approach to drug purchasing used by both the VA and the Department of Defense.

Some of the most promising changes in confronting pharmaceutical pricing have been instituted in certain states. For example, Oregon limits payment for drugs found to be ineffective. (Sounds eminently reasonable, doesn't it?) This has come to be known as *value-pricing* and is being promoted by some politicians in Washington, DC. However, that brought about debate about how value is to be measured. A range of options are on the table—years of life gained, years of life gained without disease, years of added benefit, and so on.

More aggressive enforcement of anti-trust legislation is an option that health policy analysts continue to advocate. Increased competition always seems to help keep prices under control, as it has in the case of generics. Meanwhile, major pharmaceutical companies continue to consolidate, effectively reducing the number of competitors.

If you are interested in immersing yourself in more criticism of the pharmaceutical industry, I can recommend a couple of classic reads: *The Truth About the Drug Companies* by Marcia Angell (2004) and *Our Daily Meds* by Melody Petersen (2008).

Chapter 8

Healthcare Systems in Other Countries

At this point, I'd say we are far better prepared than we were when we first started this venture to address the question of whether the claim made by many Americans—that the US healthcare system is the best in the world—is correct. The preceding chapters made clear that our system has some serious problems. But you might say that other countries' healthcare systems are not perfect either. That is, of course, very true. People in every country have complaints. Still, looking at some basic objective measures, many countries clearly do a much better job delivering healthcare services to their populations than we do.

This chapter takes a closer look at the healthcare delivery systems in the four countries we looked at in the first chapter, plus three others. Descriptions of each system begin with World Bank statistics on life expectancy and expenditures based on World Health Organization (WHO) data collected in 219 countries in 2019. Satisfaction ratings published by Statista are included for the countries it has surveyed.[1] Comparable statistics for the United States appear in each case.

Let's begin with Canada and the United Kingdom because, as mentioned in the first chapter, when people in the United States talk about healthcare systems in other countries, these are the two countries that get the most attention. It is not unusual to hear folks in this country say the Canadian and UK systems are socialistic. This is, of course, meant to invoke images of failure, grinding bureaucracy, and incompetence. However, people in both Canada and the United Kingdom live longer, pay less for health care, and express greater satisfaction with their healthcare systems. That is hard to ignore.

We turn next to the health systems in Switzerland and Japan because, as also mentioned in the first chapter, the two countries have, for some time, been recognized as having the longest life expectancy in the world. Three other countries—Spain, France, and Germany—come under review in this chapter for very specific reasons: the Spanish system because of Spain's sudden rise to fourth place in life expectancy according to the WHO; the French system because the OECD nominated it as the best healthcare system in the world, a designation which received a great deal of attention at the time and drew attention to the criteria on which it was based; and the German system because of its status as the oldest healthcare system in Europe.

CANADA

Canadians live to 82.8 years of age and spend 10.8 percent of GDP on health care; 46 percent say they are very or mostly satisfied with the healthcare system. (By comparison, Americans live to 78.2 years, spend 16.78 percent of GDP, and have a 30 percent satisfaction rate.)

Canada is made up of thirteen governmental entities: ten provinces, which are like our states but more independent of the federal government than American states, and three territories (the Yukon Territory, the Northwest Territories, and Nunavut). The Canadian healthcare system got its start in 1867 with the passage of the British North American Act, which gave the federal government responsibility for marine hospitals and the right to institute quarantines. This part of the law is comparable to the legislation passed in the United States establishing the public health service. The legislation also authorized provincial/territorial governments to assume responsibility for hospitals, asylums, charities, and charitable institutions.

The first significant step in the development of the Canadian healthcare system occurred when one of the western provinces, Saskatchewan, established a hospital insurance plan in 1947. The federal government responded by passing legislation in 1957 encouraging the creation of hospital insurance programs nationwide. By 1961, all the provinces had signed on. Once this happened, the federal government agreed to pay half the cost. The financial windfall of federal support for hospital insurance led Saskatchewan to create a medical insurance program to cover physicians' fees. Saskatchewan physicians had not been happy about the hospital plan. They were far more unhappy about the medical portion of the plan. They staged a twenty-three-day strike across the province, arguing that this was the beginning of socialized medicine, which would cause quality to decline, costs to go up because of mismanagement, and treatments to be determined by bureaucrats. The citizens of the province thought otherwise. Saskatchewan introduced medical insurance in 1961. The other provinces followed. And by 1971, Canada had a National Health Insurance Program called Medicare.

The circumstances underlying Saskatchewan citizens' willingness to consider establishing a provincial hospital plan are worth examining more closely. This is a wheat-growing province. For all you city dwellers, what do you think the growers do with the wheat they harvest? They don't take it to the local grocery store or farmers' market to sell it. It has to be processed. And they don't install a wheat-processing plant in their backyards. Even if they could process it themselves, how would they organize packaging it and selling it, getting bids on it outside of their own community, delivering it, and so on? The way this works is that growers in each community got together long ago to create cooperative processing plants. The plants then sell the processed wheat to wholesalers, who buy from many similar co-ops and sell it, in bulk, to companies that make bakery products, cereals, and so on. Now here is the critical point. The co-op pays growers based on the weight of the wheat they bring in. All the growers are closely involved in co-op operations because their livelihood depends on how well it functions. They track how much wheat sells for in international markets; they determine who serves as co-op manager; they decide whether the equipment needs to be replaced or repaired; and so on.

Does that help explain why a hospital insurance plan to which everyone would contribute and which would cover everyone in the province developed here? Not to belabor the point, but the citizens of Saskatchewan had experience working together to establish a well-functioning cooperative arrangement in which everyone was willing to participate. This provided the foundation for trust in the arrangements the members of the community established to carry out a critical function, the provision of healthcare services. Extending this account, what does the fact that the other provinces were quick to adopt both hospital and medical insurance tell you about Canadians? I would suggest it reflects confidence in the ability of the provincial government to take on responsibility for something as important as access to health care. Yes, there was some opposition, but you have to admit that they succeeded in working that out and passed the legislation at rocket speed compared to how long it is taking the United States to provide health insurance coverage for everyone in the country.

The Canada Health Act of 1984 finalized arrangements by consolidating the two earlier pieces of legislation. It made clear that provincial health plans would have to observe five principles. They would have to be: 1) publicly administered, 2) comprehensive, 3) universal, 4) portable across all provinces, and 5) accessible, in other words, with no added fees.

The Canadian Medicare plan is generally referred to as a "single-payer" plan. The single-payer is, of course, the government. Although coverage must be comprehensive, additional services, such as dental benefits, home care, and drugs, are offered at the discretion of the province. In other words, the plans differ across provinces. Insurance offered by private insurance companies is legal to cover any services a province does not provide. About two-thirds of the population has some form of private insurance, primarily for covering drug costs.

The majority of hospitals are privately owned and operated by nonprofit organizations. Most doctors are paid on a fee-for-service basis, although some opt to be paid on a salaried basis by the hospitals with which they are associated. Patients are free to choose any primary care doctor they want. Canadians are issued a Medicare card, like a credit card. Doctors' and hospital charges are reimbursed directly by the government, so patients receive no bills.

Hospitals receive a fixed amount of money on an annual basis that covers basic operating expenses plus inflation but must negotiate any major expenses separately. The state of the province's finances and the position taken by its political leadership determine how generous the province is in agreeing to fund additional hospital expenditures for technology and other kinds of upgrades.

It is not unusual to hear Americans say the Canadian system is not serving its citizens well. Just look at how many come to the United States for medical care, they say. Consider the 2020 Statista survey indicating that when Canadians were asked whether they were satisfied or dissatisfied with their healthcare arrangement: 46 percent said they were very or fairly satisfied. Only 26 percent said they were not very or not at all satisfied. That is nearly the reverse of what Americans said about our system: 43 percent of Americans said they were not very or not at all satisfied, and only 30 percent were very or fairly satisfied.

What about all those Canadians who come here to get health care? The answer is they come because this country is willing to allow anyone who can pay for the privilege to get healthcare services on demand. The vast majority come because this country permits them to get to the head of the line if they're willing to pay for it.

Canadian patients do not refer themselves to specialists. They see family practitioners for routine care who refer them to specialists when they determine this to be necessary. Physicians' fees are generally reimbursed in full for all the charges they submit. Why doesn't this result in unlimited charges? Because the annual budget is capped. Physician fee schedules are determined through negotiation between each respective provincial government and provincial medical society. The provincial government generally doesn't run out of funds for the year because it budgets what it will spend based on the record of expenditures over the previous year and the revenue it expects to collect.

However, there have been occasions when a province has run out of money, as happened in 2004 in Ontario, the richest province. When they were told the province was running out of funds for the year, physicians agreed to accept 75 percent of the scheduled fee after reaching $465,000. That might not strike you as a big sacrifice, but it's not something that doctors or anyone else would be likely to do in this country if the state was about to run out of money—now is it?

As an aside, states in this country are prohibited from ending the fiscal year with debt, which the federal government regularly does, and then goes on to raise the debt ceiling. States do run out of funds sometimes but manage to balance their budgets at the end of the year anyway. They accomplish this by putting off paying their bills. Delaying Medicaid payments to doctors and hospitals until the following year has been a common tactic. If the state's finances do not improve, the state repeats the pattern the following year, possibly over multiple years. This practice is not as common today as it was in the past.

American physicians have traditionally considered the Canadian reimbursement arrangement in which the government plays a significant role to be unacceptable. Canadian physicians see it as preferable to the constant "micromanagement" that American physicians put up with from insurance companies, pointing out that American physicians have to get preapproval from patients' insurance companies to make sure the insurance plan covers the procedure so that they will be paid for performing it and the patient will not end up being billed. Because there are so many plans with so many variations in coverage with rules that may change at any time, doctors cannot easily avoid this step. Physicians and a few medical professional organizations in this country periodically issue statements indicating support for the Canadian single-payer approach.

Canadian physicians are willing to accept a negotiated fee schedule because of two notable differences in expenses faced by Canadian physicians in contrast to American physicians. American doctors typically enter into practice with a large educational debt. Canadian medical schools are heavily subsidized by the government, meaning that medical school tuition is currently about $11,000 or so per year (in US dollars), depending on the province. This is in sharp contrast to how much American medical education costs. The second difference between Canadian and US arrangements has to do with malpractice insurance, which is much lower in Canada. This is mainly because contingency fees are considered unethical or illegal. (Remember, the contingency fee that goes to lawyers in this country is generally a third or a quarter of the settlement, depending on whether the case is settled in or out of court, and there is no fee if they lose the case.)

Canadians find themselves periodically arguing about the performance of their healthcare system because the provinces have, from time to time, had to decide whether to come up with additional funding or cut services. The federal contribution to healthcare costs, which was 50 percent originally, was cut severely during the 1980s and frozen during the 1990s when Canada experienced a recession. It was raised from 14 percent to 16 percent in 2003. Minor annual adjustments brought it up to 22 percent as of 2020.

As you can imagine, talking about compensating for a drop in federal funding has repeatedly fired up public debate about where the necessary funds will come from. At the same time, polls have long found Canadians expressing strong support for maintaining the single-payer arrangement, meaning they overwhelmingly reject two-tier care and user fees for core services. They take the position that anything not accessible to the entire population violates the spirit of the law that created the Canadian Medicare system.

We have a lot in common with Canadians. We share a very lengthy border. We speak the same language. We have similar historical roots. People in other countries can't tell us apart. So, if we are so much like them and their healthcare arrangements produce superior outcomes—they spend less than we do, everyone is fully covered by health insurance, they live a little longer than we do, and they seem to be quite satisfied—why don't we just copy it and be done with it? The answer is that no matter how alike we appear on the outside, the Canadian plan reflects their values, which are not our values. Even if some people in this country would like the United States to embrace their values, that is not how it works. Consider some of the objections heard in this country.

In the Canadian system, everyone is covered by the same plan, which means you cannot buy more, faster, or better care. Americans refuse to accept that kind of arrangement. Most Canadians take the position that "when everyone is in the same boat, that boat is likely to be much better cared for." In other words, it is always easier to deny funding to "them," but when it is "us" whose care is at stake, "we" tend to exhibit more concern and readiness to treat the topic of the need for increased funding more seriously.

To sum up, the most important differences between the Canadian system and ours are that theirs is a single-payer, capped system, while ours depends on market forces and competition to control costs; theirs provides healthcare coverage for everyone, ours does not; theirs costs less than ours; and it's hard to question quality of care since they live longer than we do. This, of course, just scratches the surface of things that people can argue about in discussing the differences between the Canadian system and the US system.

ENGLAND

People in England live to 82.2 years of age and spend 10.15 percent of GDP on health care. (Americans live to age 78.2 and spend 16.78 percent of GDP on health care.) We'll turn to satisfaction in a moment.

England, Scotland, Wales, and Northern Ireland make up the United Kingdom. Because the healthcare systems are not identical throughout the United Kingdom, the following discussion focuses on England, where health insurance for workers came into existence around 1911. Employers did not consider the health of the rest of the family to be their responsibility. The logic is clear. Remember, England was the place the industrial revolution began. The industrialists were interested in making sure their workers were healthy. Their main concern was workforce stability, not anyone's health per se, and certainly not the health of persons who were not their employees.

The history of hospital development in England serves as a particularly graphic illustration of how social values influence the character of the country's social institutions.[2] Hospitals were established several centuries ago (some as early as the sixteenth and seventeenth centuries) with the express purpose of serving three separate segments of the population. The aristocracy went to sanatoriums located in the countryside, where the patients could benefit from clean air and the special comforts the rich expected. The working poor (i.e., all workers, in contrast to the aristocracy who do not hold down jobs to this day) went to voluntary hospitals often operated by religious orders. That left the "undeserving poor" (i.e., those who were too sick, too old, too disabled, or unable to work for other reasons). Because the aristocracy would not mix with the working poor and neither would mix with the undeserving poor, each segment had to have its own hospital. All that changed with World War II.

During the war, the government mapped out all the hospitals, counted all the hospital beds in the country, and mandated that 10 percent of the beds in each hospital be set aside for military use, abolishing the differences across the three types of hospitals. The hospitals were paid a *per diem* (daily) rate whether the bed was in use or not. Everyone in the country was making sacrifices. This was the hospitals' contribution to the war effort. While the country came out of the war victorious, it sustained heavy damage and was broke. The government proposed taking over responsibility for the entire healthcare system as a reward to the public for making enormous sacrifices during wartime. In other words, from then on, the government took over the whole healthcare system. Not everyone was entirely happy about this plan. Doctors were especially loud in their objections. They said the government's plan was socialized medicine and would bring with it the downfall of professional medical practice. Looking at it objectively, it was, for better or worse, a major step toward socialized medicine. Doctors objected to being salaried instead of being paid as professionals under the traditional fee-for-service arrangement. Still, one has to be practical in these matters. Having the government provide a guaranteed income was not easy to dismiss, given the postwar state of affairs.

The solution was interesting. The general practitioners agreed to be paid under a *capitation* arrangement. They acceded to having X number of patients (around 2,000 depending on whether the practice was in an urban or rural area) sign up with them for care and get paid "by the head," whether those patients came to see them or not. This meant that doctors were guaranteed a steady income. The patients were guaranteed the services of a doctor. Patients could change doctors once a year by signing up with a new doctor of their choice. The specialists made a different bargain. They agreed to be salaried and work for a particular hospital in return for having access to 10 percent of the beds in that hospital for their private patients, whom they could bill separately. Everyone else working in the hospital had always been salaried, so that did not change.

In short, England has had a National Health Service, the NHS (not a national health insurance system), since 1948, with everyone in the country having full access to healthcare services. In assuming responsibility for the hospitals starting in 1948, the government took over ownership of all the hospitals and clinics and paid everyone who worked for the NHS.

What you hear in this country is that the Brits have to wait for an unreasonable amount of time to receive the services they need, especially high-tech tests such as CT scans, MRIs, and surgery. So, they must be registering unhappiness, right? That's not what the data show. According to 2019 Statista data, 53 percent of Brits said they were very or fairly satisfied with their healthcare arrangements, and only 22 percent said they were not very or not at all satisfied. (The American figures are 30 percent satisfied and 43 percent dissatisfied.)

Further evidence of how the Brits feel about the NHS was documented in a 2014 survey indicating that it outranks the monarchy in popularity. The monarchy has been very popular for historical and symbolic reasons. That was certainly true as long as Queen Elizabeth II reigned.[3] The Brits also exhibited a very public display of affection for the NHS during the 2012 Olympics.

A more concrete way of assessing satisfaction is to count how many people opt out of the system. That is, how many Brits choose to buy private insurance and opt to go to private doctors and hospitals? Until the 1980s, only about 5 percent of the population chose to buy private insurance. Currently, about 11 percent purchase it. What advantage are people seeking in buying private insurance if they have access to free care? Better doctors, better technology, and/or more care? Not exactly. The answer is—getting around the "queue," in other words, to avoid waiting in line for particular tests and treatments. To keep costs down, the NHS prevents people from getting healthcare services "on-demand" (i.e., whenever they feel like it) for problems that are not life-threatening. In other words, people must wait while more urgent cases get attention first. Those who think the wait is too long and can afford to do so buy private insurance and seek care in private hospitals. One of the most often-cited reasons for doing this has been hip replacement surgery. It is painful but not life-threatening.

It is important to understand another feature of how this works. Should something go seriously wrong at the private hospital, the patient is picked up by ambulance and taken to a major NHS hospital equipped to deal with high-risk and complicated problems.

People buy private insurance because the government keeps the budget for the NHS low—much too low, in the opinion of some. (England has been spending a little less than half of what we spend, as reflected in the percentage of GDP.) In theory, the Brits could change this. After all, it is their social institution; they created it, and they can change it, right? That is true. But remember, this is the NHS, not a public insurance plan. Its budget is in the hands of the ruling political party heading up the government.

Because people must weigh their dissatisfaction with the way the government is treating one social institution against how they think it is treating other social institutions, they may not be so eager to oust the current political party until they are unhappy enough about all of it. That does happen, but they are more apt to try to convince the government via appeals and protests first.

The Conservative Party, in office during the 1980s, impressed with US efforts to introduce competition to increase efficiency, created a mechanism to promote greater efficiency, known as "fund holding." This gave general practitioners the option of managing their own funds and spending the money they saved in running the practice on anything the practice group wanted to purchase. (They could not keep the surplus as a bonus.) Policymakers were somewhat surprised to find that the groups used the funds to ensure that social services were more closely aligned with medical services. The American way would have been to spend it on high-tech equipment and to build impressive new facilities to attract more patients—right? It just goes to show how cultural values shape social institutions and how they vary from one country to another.

By the end of the 1990s, the shift to a Labour Government introduced many changes the population was clamoring for. New diagnostic and treatment facilities were built to reduce waiting times. A National Institute for Clinical Excellence was established and mandated to issue binding recommendations regarding the delivery of medical services funded by the NHS. Doctors were now required to go through re-licensure every five years. As of April 2004, general practitioners were permitted to choose among a number of contractual incentive arrangements for the first time, including incentives for reaching particular service targets, for example, a higher vaccination rate. This was part of an effort to reach ten specific quality improvement targets, reducing cancer deaths by 20 percent. Contracts with specialists, called "consultants," changed only to the extent that NHS patients were now permitted, for the first time, to schedule their own appointments with specialists online.

The election of a Conservative-led coalition government in 2010 brought about a new wave of sweeping changes. Hospitals were encouraged to separate from the NHS and become independent nonprofit organizations. General practitioners (GPs) were given far more authority and funds to negotiate for services to be delivered by hospitals. GPs did not exactly welcome the changes. They said they did not believe they had the administrative background to take on this kind of responsibility and risk, nor did they have any desire to do so. Others said that they expected administrative costs to increase rather than decrease in response to this change, using the high administrative costs associated with competition in the United States to make the point.

While the public may be reasonably satisfied with the NHS, doctors in training, known as "junior doctors," are very dissatisfied these days. They went on strike at the end of 2022 because the government gave a raise to senior doctors but not to them. They say that they cannot manage on the amount they are paid. Doctors' strikes are not unusual in the United Kingdom.

What is clear about how the NHS operates is that the political party in office is in a position to make changes in the country's healthcare arrangements. This means that some people will like the changes and others will not. But one thing does not change—everyone continues to have full health insurance coverage, which may explain why most Brits are far more satisfied with their arrangements than we are.

SWITZERLAND

The Swiss live to 84.3 years of age and spend 11.3 percent of GDP on health care. (Americans live to age 78.2 and spend 16.78 percent of GDP on health care. The Swiss satisfaction rate is unavailable.)

During the two years before the Affordable Care Act (ACA) was passed, politically conservative health policy types in the United States campaigned to have the United States adopt the Swiss system. The feature they liked most was that the Swiss were expected to purchase health insurance on an individual basis from private sector companies.

A closer look at how the Swiss plan evolved and how it operates reveals that the freedom to choose one's own health insurance plan is more constrained than it first appears.[4] The system underwent significant reform in 1996 when the purchase of health insurance became compulsory for everyone in the country—at birth. The country has had universal health insurance coverage from that time forward. What spurred the reform was public opposition to the fact that women were being charged more for insurance coverage. The reform meant everyone would pay the same premium for a basic plan. A government committee determines what services will be covered. Premium prices vary based on how high the deductible is for a particular plan. The committee in charge of mandating services relies heavily on evidence-based research, often research conducted in other countries.

The system is closely monitored by the government. The enforcement of the individual mandate makes that clear. Every individual must register or be registered with the canton in which they reside—at birth. There are twenty-six cantons responsible for licensing providers, hospital planning, and subsidizing those who need help paying for insurance. If an individual does not purchase insurance coverage, the canton selects a plan for that person and bills the person or person's family in the case of children.

Health reform advocates in the United States were forced to reconsider their support for the Swiss plan once more information came out. The Swiss system includes a variety of copayments for routine medical care, drugs, and hospital stays. That means the Swiss pay for about 20 percent of their health-care out-of-pocket. Americans pay about 11.6 percent and consider this to be much too high. The Swiss system was a nonstarter once American policymakers learned how much the Swiss were paying out-of-pocket.

JAPAN

The Japanese live to 84.8 years of age, spend 10.74 percent of GDP on health care, and have a 35 percent satisfaction rate. (The US figures are: 78.2 years of age, 16.78 percent, and 30 percent.)

US health policymakers do not consider the Japanese system a good model because Japanese culture differs so much from Western culture, as represented in their diet, music, art, religion, and so on. However, since the Japanese have had the longest or near-longest life expectancy among leading economically advanced countries for the past several decades, exploring how much their healthcare system has to do with it has attracted the interest of American health policy analysts.

And no, it's not because of their diet. Once you start looking into behavior, you find that, yes, their diet is healthier because it involves less fat and carbohydrates, but some other behaviors are not as healthy. For example, they smoke far more than Americans do, at least men do. One other aspect related to behavior—homicide—offers a critical insight that explains a lot about both their health status and expenditures. The Japanese homicide rate is virtually nonexistent compared to ours.

Without getting too sidetracked by this topic, it is worth noting that the 2020 CIA World Fact Book report on homicide indicates that Japan's homicide rate per 100,000 persons was zero. You might also be interested to know that the Swiss rate was one per 100,000 persons, while the US rate was seven per 100,000 persons. Centers for Disease Control (CDC) data reveals that the homicide rate for 2022 is 7.5 per 100,000, with 5.9 of those due to firearms. And firearms are the leading cause of death for pregnant women. It is estimated that treating people affected by violence added $429 million in direct medical costs in 2017—at the acute stage.[5] There is no estimate of how much it adds for the treatment that follows over victims' lifetimes.

The history of Japanese health insurance arrangements goes back to 1927 when Japan mandated that companies employing ten or more persons provide employer-based health insurance. Currently, 59 percent of the population is covered by employment-based plans. There are over 1,400 plans to which both employees and employers contribute. They may be self-funded by employers or government-managed and partially government-subsidized.

Persons not in the labor force may or may not have had coverage depending on where they lived until 1961 when the government required municipalities to provide health insurance for anyone not covered by employer-based insurance. Japan has had universal coverage since then. Residence-based plans cover those under 75 years of age who are not insured by an employer (i.e., 27 percent of the population). Insurance for the Elderly Plans cover those over seventy-five years of age. The country is organized into forty-seven prefectures and 1,700 municipalities. Each prefecture is required to create a cost-control plan. The government closely monitors all plans.

Americans find Japanese healthcare arrangements very different from ours. Another aspect of their culture, with its accompanying set of beliefs, accounts for how they manage to spend so much less. They have about one-third less surgery than we do because organ replacement is culturally unacceptable and restricted by law. The fact that Japan built its healthcare system by grafting Western medical practices onto a system based on oriental, basically Chinese, medicine accounts for the Japanese attitude regarding surgery. Many Japanese doctors advocate the use of herbal medications as well as pharmaceuticals used in Western medicine. They not only prescribe but dispense both kinds of medications. To put this into context, oriental medicine favors medication and discourages surgery. So, there is a lot of prescribing.

The Japanese are, however, very enthusiastic about one form of Western medicine, namely, diagnostic procedures. As you may recall from chapter 1, they have many CT scanners and machines than other economically advanced countries.

It is also true that Japan has been reluctant to lower hospital costs by reducing the length of hospital stays. Japanese patients stay in the hospital far longer than Americans do—during the mid-1990s, the US average length of stay was 5.1 days, while the Japanese stay ranged from 15.8 to 29.1 days, depending on the hospital. This is explained, in part, by the fact that the Japanese have not been ready to build nursing homes for extended-stay patients. This is still a far more traditional society than ours, where women have historically stayed home and cared for aging parents and sick relatives. Even though more women have entered the labor force, the healthcare delivery system has been slow to catch up. People have dealt with the change in women's roles by checking in their elderly relatives for an extended stay when caring for the aging relative got too burdensome or when they went on vacation.

In the spring of 2000, the government agreed to do something about the problem. It passed legislation funding long-term care for the elderly. However, the number of nursing homes ready to accept elderly patients has not expanded rapidly. Japanese society continues to be reluctant to institutionalize elderly relatives for more than limited periods. The shift in attitude and behavior was expected to move forward slowly, making the transition socially and financially manageable.

SPAIN

The Spanish live to 83.9 years of age and spend 9.13 percent of GDP, with a 43 percent satisfaction rate. (The US figures are: 78.2 years of age, 16.78 percent, and 30 percent.)

The Spanish healthcare system evolved much later than in other European countries. Spain was considered an underdeveloped country ruled by a dictator, General Franco, until he died in 1975. This is when Spain suddenly became a democracy. It instituted a new constitution making health care a right in 1978. In 1986, it passed The National Health Care Act, which established seventeen Autonomous Committees charged with managing regional healthcare arrangements, which operate under the authority of the Ministry of Health. This is a single-payer arrangement. All healthcare workers, including physicians, are salaried. Hospitals are both private and public; however, public hospitals have more beds. The government covers 70 percent of healthcare costs. The cost of dental and eye care is not covered. Private insurance, which 15 percent of the population has, can be used to cover the cost of anything that is not covered, as well as basic health services.

FRANCE

The French live to 83.2 years of age, spend 11.1 percent of GDP on health care, and register a 47 percent satisfaction rate. (The US figures are: 78.2 years of age, 16.78 percent, and 30 percent.)

Although US policymakers are not interested in debating the strengths and weaknesses of the French system, the fact that the OECD nominated it as the best healthcare system in the world comes up regularly, even though that happened years ago in 2008. This was in recognition that France had the lowest number of preventable deaths compared to other economically advanced countries. The OECD has offered updated assessments, but for some reason, they have not attracted nearly as much attention, which is not to say the measure is being ignored.

The evolution of the French health insurance system began in 1945, when coverage for employees and retirees was mandated. The mandate was extended to the self-employed in 1966 and the unemployed in 2000. France has had universal coverage since that time. Health insurance is compulsory, offered by forty-two non-competitive health insurance funds. Payroll taxes provide 53 percent of the funding; employers pay 80 percent of the payroll tax, and employees pay the rest. A national earmarked income tax covers 34 percent of national healthcare expenditures. Other taxes contribute to the remaining 12 percent. Individuals are permitted to purchase supplementary insurance on top of the basic plan through their employers or private companies.

The government has been increasingly involved in controlling healthcare costs. It regulates about 75 percent of healthcare expenditures. It oversees policy for public health and the organization and financing of the healthcare system by budgeting expenditures for hospitals, ambulatory care, mental health, services for the disabled, and regions of the country.[6]

GERMANY

Germans live to 81.0 years of age and spend 11.7 percent of GDP. (The US figures are: 78.2 years of age and 16.78 percent; the German satisfaction is unavailable.)

The German healthcare system is the oldest national healthcare system in Europe. It was introduced in 1871 by Otto von Bismarck, prime minister of a section of Germany—Prussia—who reasoned that if workers thought the government was meeting their needs, they would be less likely to support radical political movements permitting his government to stay in control.

The system took shape in 1883 with the passage of the Sickness Insurance Act, which required all workers below a certain income level to join existing mutual benefit societies. The societies, created by guilds and villages to help cover unanticipated costs, such as funerals and lost income resulting from temporary injuries or permanent disability, had existed for two or three hundred years. Over time, they developed units to deal with health care called "sickness funds."

The development of the German system has some peculiar historical features that are interesting to reflect on. For example, the 1883 law gave sickness funds the authority to operate health clinics and hire doctors. Because the sickness funds were small and run by persons who didn't necessarily have the skill to manage large sums of money, doctors were often not paid as promised. They responded by going out on strike whenever that happened. While doctors were very dissatisfied with prevailing arrangements, they had little influence over national healthcare arrangements because they had no professional association to represent their views. Germany's doctors did not organize themselves into a national association until 1931. (Remember, the American Medical Association came into existence in 1847.)

How doctors are paid is an interesting feature of the German system. Doctors are either office-based or hospital-based. Their practices do not overlap. The hospital-based doctors are salaried. Office-based doctors are paid on a fee-for-service basis, according to a fee schedule established in negotiations between sickness funds and physicians' groups. The fees are subject to a cap, which works in response to an interesting and effective mechanism. Medical expenditures are reviewed quarterly by the local medical society. If the total expenditure on office-based physicians' fees exceeds the projected amount, the fees for all office-based practitioners are reduced. Doctors whose fees are significantly higher than those of their colleagues then come under scrutiny—not by bureaucrats but instead by a committee of fellow physicians who have the expertise to evaluate the reasons behind the high rate and authority to impose sanctions on doctors found to be "overtreating" patients. That tends to keep the lid on medical expenditures.

The German healthcare system evolved as society modernized. The number of sickness funds declined over time as some failed and others merged. As of 2022, there are about 110 funds. High-income individuals may opt out of coverage by sickness funds. Accordingly, 88 percent of the population is covered by sickness funds, and 11 percent is covered by private insurance.

MORE ON INTERNATIONAL COMPARISONS

Many organizations and individuals are ready to offer international healthcare system ratings. This includes IBM, *U.S. News and World Report*, various health insurance companies, travel organizations, and assorted bloggers. You won't be surprised to find that they don't all agree. The difference results from the variation in indicators they choose to rely on.

The indicator that many analysts agree is important, but which gets relatively little attention, is "preventable deaths," initially used by the Organisation for Economic Co-operation and Development (OECD) to recognize France as having the best healthcare system in the world. France dropped to twelfth place on the OECD list of countries with the lowest rate of preventable deaths as of 2017. This was when Israel moved to the top of the list with seventy-two preventable deaths per 100,000 persons in the population, followed by Switzerland at eighty-five deaths and Japan at eighty-seven deaths. The United States came in near the bottom of the list with 175 preventable deaths out of 100,000 persons. The United States did a little better in terms of mortality from treatable causes, but its performance was still surpassed by twenty-seven other countries.

The OECD defines preventable death as "death that can be avoided through effective public health and prevention interventions." It defines "treatable causes of death" as "causes that can be mainly avoided through timely and effective healthcare interventions." It reports the rate of both categories among its thirty-eight member countries based on WHO data.[7] The 2017 list of causes of *preventable deaths* includes cancer (32 percent), external causes (25 percent), circulatory system (19 percent), alcohol and drug effects (9 percent), respiratory system (8 percent), and others (7 percent). The mortality from *treatable causes of death* list includes circulatory system (38 percent), cancer (28 percent), others (20 percent), respiratory system (9 percent), and diabetes/other endocrine diseases (9 percent).

If we are spending so much more on health care than other countries, why can't we do a better job of dealing with such deaths?

A 2021 report issued by the Commonwealth Fund examining the health systems in eleven high-income countries, relying on OECD and WHO data, offers a comprehensive analysis of differences across the countries, providing us with a better understanding of responsible factors.[8] The study reports on seventy-one performance indicators across five domains: access to care, care process, administrative efficiency, equity, and healthcare outcomes. The overall ranking of the effectiveness of healthcare systems in addressing mortality and morbidity based on these indicators is as follows: 1) Norway, 2) Netherlands, 3) Australia, 4) the United Kingdom, 5) Germany, 6) New Zealand, 7) Sweden, 8) France, 9) Switzerland, 10) Canada, and 11) the United States.

In explaining what distinguishes the top-performing countries, the Commonwealth Fund identifies four characteristics:

1. They provide for universal coverage and remove cost barriers;
2. They invest in primary care systems to ensure that high-value services are equitably available in all communities to all people;

3. They reduce administrative burdens that divert time, effort, and spending from health improvement efforts; and
4. They invest in social services, especially for children and working-age adults.

As to the US rating, the Commonwealth Fund report states that the United States ranks last overall, despite spending far more of its gross domestic product on health care. The United States ranks last on access to care, administrative efficiency, equity, and healthcare outcomes but second on care process measures.

SOME FINAL OBSERVATIONS

While the accounts we've just reviewed of how different countries came to have the healthcare systems they have today speak for themselves, I propose to offer a few final observations. It is clear that the countries we've discussed addressed concerns about health care at different times in their history. Once the foundations of their systems were in place, they just built on top of those foundations. Retrospectively, we can see that industrialization spurred countries like England and Germany to address the healthcare needs of workers during the late nineteenth century. The post–World War II period brought forth notable reforms in a number of other European countries. The late 1970s and early 1980s were major turning points when most European countries got their expenditures under control while expenditures in the United States continued to rise (table 8.1).

What is notable is that other countries managed to achieve that, even as they moved toward universal coverage and increased government oversight over expenditures. This is when the United States opted for a different approach. It

Table 8.1. Percent GDP spent on health care, 1970–2021

Country	1970*	1980*	1990*	2021**
Canada	7.0	7.2	9.2	12.8
France	5.8	7.6	8.9	12.2
Germany	6.3	8.8	8.7	12.8
Japan	4.6	6.5	6.1	11.1
Spain	3.7	5.6	6.9	10.7
Switzerland	4.9	6.9	8.3	11.8
United Kingdom	4.5	5.6	6.0	12.0
United States	7.3	9.1	12.6	18.8

*Manfred Huber. 1999. "Health Expenditure Trends in OECD Countries, 1970–1997." *Health Care Financing Review,* winter 21 (2): 99–117.

** "OECD Health Spending." 2021. https://data.oecd.org/healthres/health-spending.htm.

moved toward control by the private sector, together with increased reliance on consolidation, market forces, and competition.

It is fair to say that other countries support competition as long as it does not interfere with the basic healthcare plan that covers everyone in the country. And it is interesting to see how competition looks when other countries embrace it. Somehow it doesn't look much like it does in this country.

Can we, in turn, learn from the experiences of other countries? Perhaps. Americans tend toward xenophobia—we seem to have a strong need to reject what is foreign. Unlike the Europeans and Japanese, who have been importing ideas based on our experiments, we prefer to think we are better off creating new mechanisms from scratch. Health policymakers keep introducing a steady stream of mechanisms, which they are prepared to discard when the mechanisms fail to deliver what was promised. Then, they simply go on to invent and reinvent some more. Winston Churchill's oft-repeated judgment of American ingenuity may be apropos here. He is said to have observed that Americans can be counted on to make the right decision—after exhausting every other possible option. We can hope that his assessment will apply to our healthcare system—in the long run. But who knows when.

Chapter 9

Determinants of Health

Now that we've completed a thorough examination of this country's health-care arrangements, let's go full circle back to chapter 1 to ask the following: Does understanding the workings of our healthcare system explain why the United States compares so poorly to other countries when it comes to life expectancy? I will assume you don't think it does.

However, one does not have to look far for the answer. Popular culture is unrelenting in trying to convince us that our health is not as good as it could be because we're not taking care of ourselves—that we would be so much healthier if only we didn't indulge in bad habits of various kinds: eating and drinking too much, eating the wrong types of foods, not exercising, not following advice on getting better sleep, and so on. Then there are the purveyors of an endless variety of supplements promising their products will overcome much of that. And if someone indulges in bad habits their entire life and still lives to a ripe old age, we shrug and say it's genetic.

Avoiding unhealthy behaviors is certainly not a bad idea, but does personal behavior really explain why we don't live as long as people in other economically advanced countries? The World Health Organization's (WHO) stance on this topic is unequivocal in rejecting what popular culture wants us to believe.

The context of people's lives determines their health, and so blaming individuals for having poor health or crediting them for good health is inappropriate. Individuals are unlikely to be able to directly control many of the determinants of health.[1]

The social determinants of health (SDH) are the non-medical factors that influence health outcomes. They are the conditions in which people are born, grow, work, live and age and the wider set of forces and systems shaping the conditions of daily life. These forces and systems include economic policies and systems, development agencies, social norms, social policies and political systems.[2]

Before we go further, I must warn you that launching into the topic of social determinants of health won't be easy. For one, it's a topic best addressed in a full-length book rather than a single chapter. Second, it requires fortitude to confront a lot of distressing information. In the end, I expect you will find the research on social determinants of health to be eye-opening and convincing because volumes of hard data back it up. A third problem in taking up this issue is the temptation to go off on new paths of inquiry that come up throughout this discussion. I will let you know when that occurs.

The WHO provides us with a list of factors that it says play a critical role in determining people's health in order of priority. (The WHO does not use numbers; it uses bullets.)

1. Income and social status—higher income and social status are linked to better health. The greater the gap between the richest and poorest people, the greater the difference in health.
2. Education—low education levels are linked with poor health, more stress, and lower self-confidence.
3. Physical environment—safe water and clean air, healthy workplaces, safe houses, communities and roads all contribute to good health. Employment and working conditions—people in employment are healthier, particularly those who have more control over their working conditions.
4. Social support networks—greater support from families, friends, and communities is linked to better health. Culture—customs and traditions, and the beliefs of the family and community all affect health.
5. Genetics—inheritance plays a part in determining lifespan, healthiness and the likelihood of developing certain illnesses. Personal behavior and coping skills—balanced eating, keeping active, smoking, drinking, and how we deal with life's stresses and challenges all affect health.
6. Health services—access and use of services that prevent and treat disease influences health.
7. Gender—Men and women suffer from different types of diseases at different ages.[3]

Are you surprised to find that the WHO places genetics and personal behavior together with health services so far down the list, given that these are the factors that we have been repeatedly told are responsible for the state of our health? (Genetics is one of the intriguing paths we won't be running off on. It is a field of study that is much too complicated to treat as an add-on to the main topic we aim to discuss here.)

How do you feel about finding income and social status at the top of the list? That plus the idea that the greater the gap between the richest and poorest people, the greater the difference in health. As it turns out, this assessment, added to the fact that the United States has the largest gap between rich and poor across all economically advanced countries, explains a lot about what is happening in this country. The existence of tremendous economic inequality in the United States is supported by volumes of research. I refer to a small proportion of it as we move through this chapter.

A message dismissive of social inequality that I expect you will recognize is instilled in most of us from grade school on—America is the land of opportunity, and everyone can get ahead if they work at it. As a matter of fact, the United States did come closer to being the land of opportunity during the period between World War II and the 1970s. That's not the case anymore. The country has experienced a steady rise in economic inequality since then. As Joseph Stiglitz, one of this country's most highly respected economists, puts it, it is now

> one of a few developed countries jostling for the dubious distinction of having the lowest measures of equality of opportunity. . . . The life prospects of a young American depend more on the income or education of his or her parents than in almost any other advanced country. When poor-boy-makes-good anecdotes get passed around in the media, that is precisely because such stories are so rare.[4]

The reasons for the shift in opportunity are not in dispute. They include globalization and technological advancement. But all the countries to which we compare ourselves faced the same forces during the post–World War II period. They just didn't allow increasing economic inequality to take hold like we did.

As an aside, the primary reason we have so much economic inequality in this country has to do with taxation. The top tax income rate during the 1940s was 94 percent. No, that's not a typo. That's how much the people at the top of the income scale were taxed. The rate fell slowly, dropping to 50 percent in 1982 and 38.5 percent by 1987. It really dipped in 1988, down to 28 percent. It now stands at 37 percent.[5] Lowering the tax rate paid by the rich meant that people in the top income bracket were able to accumulate wealth and pass it on to the next generation, making society increasingly more unequal over time.

Clearly the differences in income from the bottom 20 percent of the population to the top 20 percent are enormous (table 9.1).

The disparity in wealth reveals a lot more (table 9.2). Just to make sure you don't miss the point: This means that 97.3 percent of the wealth in this country belongs to the top half of the population.

As an aside, the news media keeps telling us that the rich pay a far smaller percentage in taxes than the rest of us, and in some notable cases, they pay no

Table 9.1. Household income distribution for 2020, mean income by quintile

Lowest quintile	$14,500
Second quintile	$39,479
Middle quintile	$67,846
Fourth quintile	$109,732
Highest quintile	$253,284
Top 5%	$446,030

Source: Tax Policy Center, Urban Institute and Brookings Institution. (January 25, 2022) https://www
.taxpolicycenter.org/statistics/household-income-quintiles.

Table 9.2. Distribution of net wealth, 2022

90–99th percentile of the population	37.5%
50–90th percentile	27.7%
Bottom 50th percentile	2.7%
Top 1 percentile	32.2%

Source: Statista Research Department. Distribution of Wealth in the United States 1990–2022. https://www
.statista.com/statistics/299460/distribution-of-wealth-in-the-united-states/.

taxes. This can't help but confirm the existence of socioeconomic inequality. At the same time, it has not deterred others from arguing that giving the rich tax breaks is necessary because it will result in more jobs. That refrain was first popularized during the 1970s, which, not to put too fine a point on it, coincides with the unrelenting rise in socioeconomic inequality.

Okay, so there's a tremendous amount of economic inequality in this country—what does that have to do with health? It turns out it has a lot to do with health. A large number of highly respected researchers and research organizations have been paying attention. They've been tracking the pathways identified by the WHO.

I propose to focus on each of the factors identified by the WHO in the order in which they are presented, starting with education.

EDUCATION AND INEQUALITY

The research on the relationship between socioeconomic status and education and how it translates into adverse health outcomes exploded in response to a groundbreaking study of the English civil service Whitehall, conducted in two stages, beginning in 1967 and ending in 1988.[6] The basic finding was that life expectancy was directly correlated with civil service rank, which is based on educational attainment. (As an aside, in my opinion, one of the most striking findings coming out of that study was that destructive personal behavior, like smoking, was less detrimental the higher the rank.) The Whitehall studies established social inequality as the core variable explaining variation in health outcomes. Since then, volumes of follow-up research have accumulated, indicating that differences in social status have direct health consequences.[7]

The fact that people with more education live longer is indisputable. According to one group of researchers who conducted a comprehensive review of the literature on the link between education and health outcomes, about 30 percent of the correlation between education and health is explained by the economic difference it engenders.[8] The researchers outlined the mechanisms that account for this. For a start, higher education is linked to higher-paying jobs, jobs that are more secure. Job security leads to a greater chance of turning stable earnings into wealth accumulation, which, in turn, produces psychosocial security with associated health benefits.

The same researchers say that health behavior is a proximal determinant of health, meaning that better-educated people are less likely to smoke, have an unhealthy diet, and not exercise. Beyond that, the social-psychological benefits associated with education and the socioeconomic stability it provides lead to a greater chance of achieving "successful long-term marriages and other sources of social support to help cope with stressors and daily hassles."

The Council on Foreign Relations, a think tank, captures the relationship between education and economic security in table 9.3.

In presenting the data on earnings and unemployment, the Council on Foreign Relations report states that the percentage by which the wages of college graduates exceeded those of high school graduates grew rapidly from 1979 to 2000.[9] However, the advantage of getting a college degree fell appreciably after that. The authors cite a Federal Reserve study, which reported that the net worth of having a college degree declined significantly for white Americans born in the 1980s and disappeared entirely for black Americans. There are a couple of important insights here. Let's focus on the decline in the value of the college degree first and turn to race in a separate section later in this chapter.

According to the Organisation for Economic Co-operation and Development (OECD), the United States ranked first in college graduation in 1995.[10] It now

Table 9.3. Income and unemployment, 2017

Education	Weekly earnings	Unemployment rate
Professional degree	$1,836	1.5%
Bachelor's degree	$1,173	2.5%
Some college	$774	4.0%
High school	$712	4.6%
Less than high school	$520	6.5%

Source: Siripurapu, Anshu. "The U.S. Inequality Debate." Council on Foreign Relations. April 20, 2020. https://www.cfr.org/backgrounder/us-inequality-debate.

stands at nineteenth. That happened because other countries started to surpass American student achievement at a much earlier stage of education. The Pew Charitable Trusts reported on the scores achieved by fifteen-year-old students in OECD member countries in 2017 across three dimensions. US students were in twenty-fourth place in science, twenty-fourth place in reading, and thirty-eighth place in mathematics.[11]

The reason those without a college degree have been falling further behind economically is that they haven't been prepared for the shift in the types of jobs that came into existence over the last few decades of the twentieth century, jobs that require technical training grounded in basic science and mathematics. The historical context for this is important. Before the 1980s, when the US economy was based on manufacturing, unskilled workers could enter the labor force and succeed with on-the-job training. They didn't need formal education. They could move up the ladder based on what they learned on the job. They moved up the employment ladder as a steady stream of new unskilled workers entered the workforce, starting on the bottom rung of the same ladder. Job security, a stable income, and a middle-class lifestyle were possible without a college education in an industrial economy. That was true across economically advanced societies. However, other societies took steps to deal with the need to accommodate to the evolving need for a better-educated workforce. The United States did not. This has had implications for the social structure of American society.

"From 1970 to 2018, the share of aggregate income going to middle-class households fell from 62% to 48%. The share going to lower-income households inched down from 10% to 9% in 2018."[12] The result is the depletion of the middle class. With less basic education and without the necessary preparation to enter jobs requiring high-tech skills, workers whose manufacturing jobs were disappearing were thrust into the unskilled, service job market with lower wages, less job security, and fewer benefits.

DEATHS OF DESPAIR

A review of research on the negative health consequences of a high level of economic inequality and the waning middle class is summed up in a 2017 policy statement issued by the American Public Health Association.

> Countries with higher levels of income inequality have higher rates of depression, narcissism, and schizophrenia. Inequality creates frustration, stress, and a sense of being left behind, leading to lower levels of trust, happiness, and life satisfaction. The social stressors in an unequal society can drive individuals into detrimental coping mechanisms, and rates of drug and alcohol abuse,

gambling, compulsive eating, and violence are higher in unequal societies. This phenomenon is demonstrated in the drastic increase in mortality, particularly among middle-aged non-Hispanic over the past decade driven by overdoses, liver disease resulting from substance abuse, and suicide.[13]

The reference to the health outcomes exhibited by middle-aged whites brings us to a discussion of another groundbreaking report issued by two economists, Anne Case and Angus Deaton, in 2020.[14] They documented the decline in life expectancy among white working-class Americans, who they said "are drinking themselves to death, poisoning themselves with drugs, or shooting or hanging themselves." They went on to say that work that gave meaning to life, providing workers with a sense of dignity, pride, and self-respect, has disappeared. Without that, marriages failed. Unemployed men make poor husbands. Institutions that once provided community stability, such as unions and mainstream churches, no longer served that purpose. People have been looking for another way to connect, which social media was ready to provide, with what we are finding are destructive consequences. (Social media is another big topic to which we can't devote the attention it deserves.)

The statement made by Princeton University Press at Case and Deaton's book's release titled *Deaths of Despair and the Future of Capitalism* makes the following observation, one that may or may not come as a surprise to you.

In this important book, Case and Deaton tie the crisis to the weakening position of labor, the growing power of corporations, and, above all, to a rapacious healthcare sector that redistributes working-class wages into the pockets of the wealthy. Capitalism, which over two centuries lifted countless people out of poverty, is now destroying the lives of blue-collar America.[15]

The cumulative effect of rising social inequality manifests in the prevalence of deaths of despair among a large segment of the US population and has social repercussions that further exacerbate the decline in life expectancy exhibited by white working-class Americans. The American Public Health Association confirms that observation with the following assessment.

Unequal societies have decreased levels of trust and social cohesion, which fuel discontent with public institutions, increased political polarization, and sociopolitical instability. Starting in the 1970s, Americans' trust in the media, medicine, corporations, universities, and the government has steadily declined as income inequality has risen. Concomitantly, Congress has become increasingly divided and partisan, resulting in political gridlock and constituent disillusionment. Hyper-partisanship and ineffective governance further hinder efforts to mitigate the effects of income inequality on health. Without the political will to develop healthy and economically vibrant communities through investments in education, infrastructure, and social programs, communities have become geographically segregated according to income, with unequal levels of access to resources and opportunities that promote health and economic mobility. As a result, communities that lack access to high-quality education, medical care, healthy foods, and good-paying jobs are plagued by high levels of violence and incarceration, socioeconomic stagnation, and political disaffection, further hindering their ability to economically advance.[16]

As an aside, I expect that the American Public Health Association's statement may sound familiar because it sums up so well the political turmoil this country has experienced over the last few years.

In an added aside, a study across 177 countries designed to determine why some countries experienced far lower rates of Covid infections and deaths found Vietnam to have an exceptionally low rate. How was that possible in a country that scored poorly on international assessments of preparation for the pandemic? Its healthcare system was certainly not nearly as sophisticated as that of other countries. After considering a range of variables, the researchers concluded that the population had a high level of trust in its government and, so, was willing to follow instructions intended to prevent the spread of Covid.[17]

HEALTH DISPARITIES AND RACE

Black and Hispanic Americans have not suffered the same fate as working-class whites and have, in fact, enjoyed an increase in life expectancy over the last couple of decades. But this observation must be put in perspective.

> During 1999–2015, age-adjusted death rates decreased by 25 percent for blacks and 14 percent for whites. [For those over sixty-five,] there was a black-white mortality crossover, whereby blacks had slightly lower age-adjusted deaths than whites beginning in 2010. In addition, during 1999–2015, blacks saw declines in the two leading causes of death—heart disease and cancer—across all age groups. However, despite substantive reductions in death rates among blacks in the United States, blacks continue to have higher death rates overall.[18]

Not only do people of color experience higher death rates but also more troubling is finding that black and American Indian/Alaskan Native individuals are more likely to die from treatable conditions. They are more likely to die due to pregnancy-related issues and are at higher risk of chronic health conditions such as diabetes and hypertension. They are less likely to receive preventive care, such as flu shots, and more likely to seek care in an emergency room for conditions that could be managed through good primary care.

The disparity in infant mortality rates, which, as you will recall, is considered the most sensitive measure of health because it indicates the health status of the most vulnerable members of society, is staggering. It is worth stopping to reflect on the fact that the rates in these tables translate into deaths of real people, in this case, blameless infants (table 9.4).

Based on what you've read in this chapter, what do you think explains the variation in infant mortality? A lot has been written about the discrimination blacks encounter in seeking healthcare services. So, yes, we can say that it definitely plays a role.

How about personal behavior? Yes, that plays a big part too. But that, too, has to be considered in context. When the demographic characteristics of blacks and whites in this country are compared, blacks are more likely to have a lower level of education, more likely to be unemployed, live below the poverty level, and less likely to own the house they live in. They are less likely to engage in regular exercise, less likely to have a regular doctor, and those over age fifty are more likely to smoke, although less likely to smoke under the age of thirty-four.[19] Working-class middle-aged whites smoke more.

If a whole group of individuals who share certain characteristics engages in the same behavior, it's more than individual choice. The behavior is correlated with social class. Saying it is determined by social class, not by race, requires more explication. Researchers associated with the Harvard T. H. Chan School of Public Health say that racism explains the variation, that is, stress caused by persistent racial discrimination. In explaining this, they tell us they looked at a host of other possible factors for why black infant mortality is so high—such as women's poor eating habits, obesity, smoking, drinking, or poor prenatal care—but none of the factors examined, alone or together, were found to be significant to fully account for the racial gap.

Evidence now suggests that years of dealing with discrimination—living in poor, segregated neighborhoods, having to move frequently, parenting alone, or parenting with an unemployed partner—may lead to chronic stress, which

Table 9.4. Infant mortality by race and ethnicity of mother, 2020

Ethnicity	Per 1,000 live births
Black	10.58
American Indian or Alaskan Native	7.68
Native American or Pacific Islander	7.17
Hispanic	4.69
White	4.40
Asian	3.14

Source: Ely, Danielle, and Anne Driscoll. "Infant Mortality in the United States, 2020: Data From the Period Linked Birth/Infant Death File." *National Vital Statistics Report* (September 29, 2022).

takes a toll on the body and may prompt biological changes in a woman that can affect the health of her children.[20]

PHYSICAL ENVIRONMENT

Reflecting on the WHO list of factors that affect people's health, the headline of an article published by the National Community Reinvestment Coalition (NCRC) is apropos—"Your Zip Code Is More Important than Your Genetic Code."[21] It states that "up to 60% of your health is determined by your zip code."

That's understandable when you consider that one's zip code determines such health-related factors as the availability of affordable housing, good transportation, air quality, the existence of walking paths, community safety, as well as the other basic features of daily life we've already addressed, including access to good schools, food, and medical care.

Zip code serves as a "quick and dirty" indicator of the third factor on the WHO list of social determinants of health—physical environment.

SOCIAL SUPPORT NETWORKS

The fourth factor identified by the WHO is social support. The primary author associated with the Whitehall studies, Michael Marmot, has given a name to the dynamics involved—the *status syndrome*.[22] He presents us with mountains of evidence to support the ideas behind this label. Here's an enticing tidbit buried in those mountains illustrating the phenomenon. It seems that Oscar winners live four years longer than Oscar nominees who do not win the prize. The mechanism operates as follows—those who do not win compare themselves to the winner and find themselves lacking in the eyes of others and suffer the negative health consequences associated with diminished social status.

A 2022 article in the *Washington Post* concerned with friendship cites research conducted worldwide reinforcing another insight first identified by the Whitehall studies—that having more friends lowers peoples' death rates.[23] The article reports research confirming the Whitehall finding that close connections with spouses, partners, children, and other relatives do not produce the same benefit. The article includes data on the impact of social media, something the Whitehall studies did not address because it did not exist at the time. But the finding is probably something many people in this country can relate to—that social media can engender a sense of loneliness "by bombarding us with photos and videos of friends and acquaintances seemingly spending their time without us." The authors of the *Washington Post* article say it's not something people are ready to confront because loneliness has an aura of shame about it. The main idea the authors wish to convey is that the more one "hangs out" with friends, the healthier one is likely to be.

UPSTREAM VERSUS DOWNSTREAM INTERVENTION

If healthcare services and personal behavior aren't nearly as important to understanding differences in health outcomes as socioeconomic inequality, then we must look for ways to deal with poor health outcomes that take this reality into consideration. So, what do we do?

Identifying the factors primarily responsible for health disparities and doing something about them requires stepping back to adopt a new mindset. The concept embraced by the public health community for doing this involves looking *upstream* for answers.

The concept was introduced by John McKinlay, who tells the story of a physician recounting his experience of standing on the shore of a fast-flowing river and hearing the cry of a drowning man.

> So I jump in the river, put my arms around him, pull him to shore and apply artificial respiration. Just when he begins to breathe, there is another cry for help. So I jump into the river, reach him, pull him to shore, apply artificial respiration, and then just as he begins to breathe, another cry for help. So back in the river again, reaching, pulling, applying, without end, goes the sequence. You know, I am so busy jumping in, pulling them to shore, applying artificial respiration, that I have no time to see who the hell is upstream pushing them all in.[24]

Who is pushing them in? Based on what we've reviewed in this chapter, there is no question that the answer comes down to the set of forces that produce social inequality.

In recounting this tale, McKinlay makes the obvious point—we are making a huge mistake focusing on downstream efforts—that is, spending an enormous amount of money on the healthcare sector and at the same time blaming people for their health status, which in combination, prevents us from focusing on the real factors responsible for poor health outcomes.

McKinlay, along with many others, argues that society is allowing the manufacturers of illness to cause illness and death. He nominates companies that promote "illness-inducing behaviors" such as smoking, eating fatty foods, and readiness to take up guns. (Gun violence, a topic we touched on in the preceding chapter, deserves much more attention than we can devote to it here.) Case and Deaton, the economists who gained renown for their analysis of deaths of despair, blame capitalism gone awry and the rapacious healthcare industry in particular. Other economists and political scientists argue that capitalists at the top of the income and wealth ladder have created a feedback loop to shape the connection between money and regulations.[25] The loop has led to the concentration of market power in the hands of a few global players who employ social media to promote messages that serve their purpose. (Again, how social media operates to achieve this is a topic that requires a great deal more analysis.)

What is curious is finding that the organizations promoting health-damaging personal behavior are ready to turn around and blame the people who engage in that behavior for health outcomes resulting from that behavior. They are adamant about people's right to choose the behavior they engage in, even if it is self-destructive or socially destructive. They say that personal behavior is a matter of individual rights, and those rights must be protected. Any effort on the part of the government to contain behaviors destructive to health is defined as a plot designed to take away individual rights and freedoms. The advocates of the individual choice ideology have clearly had tremendous success promoting their message.

Commitment to the protection of individual rights has done little for those who experience a loss in status and economic security, plus the accompanying feelings of hopelessness. We see these people experiencing diminished social status and economic insecurity faced with choosing between two alternatives. There are those who choose to *fight* and those who turn to *flight*. The choice of the fight option, that is, resorting to violence in attacking others, accounts for this country's high homicide rate; the flight option shows up in the attempt to escape reality, as indicated by high addiction and suicide rates. (I realize these options bring us back not only to violence but also mental health issues, but that's for another book.) The choice of either the fight or flight response has devasting health consequences, even as the beneficiaries of social inequality condemn the behavior while arguing for addressing it—downstream.

The majority of Americans agree that reducing social inequality is important. As we would all concur, this is a monumental challenge to take on. The lack of agreement on who should take responsibility for it makes it so much harder to tackle. The difficulty is grounded in the fact that nominating who should do it differs depending on peoples' political affiliation and the beliefs underlying that political affiliation. This is made explicit by a Pew survey conducted in 2020.[26] The survey results indicate that 61 percent of Americans say there is too much social inequality; that breaks down into 78 percent of Democrats and 41 percent of Republicans. A far greater percentage of Republicans (60 percent) believe that inequality is due to personal behavior than Democrats (27 percent); similarly, more Republicans think hard work overcomes inequality (48 percent) than Democrats (22 percent). Those differences tie in with who they think should address the issue. A majority of Democrats say the federal government should assume responsibility (75 percent); far fewer Republicans say that (44 percent). There's also a significant difference in the proportion of Republicans who believe raising taxes on the rich is a good idea (65 percent) as opposed to the proportion of Democrats who think that's a good idea (91 percent).

The explanation for the variation in who should take responsibility has to do with the level of trust in government. In 1958, 73 percent of Americans said they trusted the US government.[27] By 2022, that dropped to 20 percent. But it's worse than that when you consider the divide by political party affiliation. While it's bad enough that only 29 percent of Democrats express trust in government, only 9 percent of Republicans do so.

A recent United Nations report reinforces everything we've learned about the role economic inequality plays in this country but goes further. The report asserts that "runaway inequality is destabilizing the world's democracies."[28] It does so by eroding trust in democratic institutions and paving the way for populist regimes. The authors point out that economic elites throughout the world aren't interested in challenging this trend because populists do not threaten the balance of power the elites enjoy. The UN report states that the history of populist regimes is characterized by corruption, self-dealing, worsening inequality, and political violence. We see ample evidence of that in this country and elsewhere.

The proposals, summed up by the Council on Foreign Relations, speak to these observations. Aimed at reducing social inequality and overcoming all the problems it presents, the proposals offered by the Council on Foreign Relations center on a more progressive income tax, a higher minimum wage, and expanded educational opportunities. Sounds reasonable, doesn't it, or does it?

FINAL THOUGHTS

We started this venture with a focus on the healthcare system, and here we are, ending up focusing on the worldwide threat to democracy. Recognizing that poor health outcomes are part of a much bigger picture requires understanding the reasons behind the factors that brought us to this point. That means we must acknowledge that improving health outcomes requires a lot more than fiddling with third-party reimbursement arrangements and some of the other policies people with good intentions propose. I'm not suggesting that health policymakers abandon such measures. Rather, I am suggesting that health policymakers take a broader view of our healthcare arrangements and, even more importantly, bring the public along with them to take in that picture. Accomplishing that constitutes an overwhelming challenge in the face of major obstacles which explains why it's not happening with any speed.

Notes

CHAPTER 1

1. "Listening to the WHO: How to Assess Health System Performance." 2002. Commonwealth Fund. Accessed January 26, 2023. https://www.linkedin.com/pulse/listening-who-how-assess-health-system-performance-/.

CHAPTER 2

1. Schneider, Mary-Jane, with Henry Schneider. 2021. *Introduction to Public Health, 6th ed.* Burlington, MA: Jones and Bartlett Learning LLC.

2. US Department of Health and Human Services. n.d. Health and Human Services Agencies and Offices. Accessed June 5, 2023. https://www.hhs.gov/about/agencies/hhs-agencies-and-offices/index.html.

3. National Association of County and City Officials. n.d. "Developing a Local Health Department Strategic Plan: A How-To Plan." Accessed December 6, 2022. https://www.naccho.org/uploads/downloadable-resources/Programs/Public-Health-Infrastructure/StrategicPlanningGuideFinal.pdf.

4. Centers for Disease Control and Prevention. n.d. "The Public Health System & the 10 Essential Public Health Services." Accessed December 1, 2022. https://www.cdc.gov/publichealthgateway/publichealthservices/essentialhealthservices.html.

5. Department of Health and Human Services, Office of Disease Prevention and Health Promotion. n.d. "History of Healthy People." Accessed November 23, 2022. https://health.gov/our-work/national-health-initiatives/healthy-people/about-healthy-people/history-healthy-people.

6. Health.gov. n.d. "History of Healthy People." Accessed February 24, 2023. https://health.gov/our-work/national-health-initiatives/healthy-people/about-healthy-people/history-healthy-people.

7. Office of the Assistant Secretary of Health. n.d. "Healthy People 2020 An End of Decade Snapshot." Accessed November 22, 2022. https://health.gov/sites/default/files/2020-12/HP2020EndofDecadeSnapshot.pdf.

8. Kreiger, Nancy, et al. 2022. "Relationship of Political Ideology of U.S. Federal and State Elected Officials and Key Covid Pandemic Outcomes Following Vaccine Rollout to Adults: April 2021–March 2022." *Lancet.* Accessed November 3, 2022. https://www.thelancet.com/journals/lanam/article/PIIS2667-193X(22)00201-0/fulltext.

9. Gaba, Charles. 2022. "September Update: Covid Death Rates by Partisan Lean & Vaccination Rate." *ACASignups.net* blog. Accessed September 11, 2022. https://acasignups.net/22/09/11/september-update-covid-death-rates-partisan-lean-vaccination-rate.

10. Kupferschmidt, Kai. 2022. "Monkeypox Cases Are Plummeting. Scientists Are Debating Why." *Science.* Accessed October 26, 2022. https://www.science.org/content/article/monkeypox-cases-are-plummeting-scientists-are-debating-why.

11. Berglas, Nancy, et al. 2018. "State and Local Health Department Activities Related to Abortion: A Web Site Content Analysis." *Journal of Public Health Management and Practice* Accessed November 21, 2022. https://journals.lww.com/jphmp/fulltext/2018/05000/state_and_local_health_department_activities.10.aspx.

12. Brennan Center for Justice, Center for Reproductive Rights. 2023. "State Court Abortion Litigation Tracker." Accessed February 24, 2023. https://www.brennancenter.org/our-work/research-reports/state-court-abortion-litigation-tracker.

13. Artiga, Samantha, et al. 2022. "What Are the Implications of Overturning Roe v Wade for Racial Disparities?" Kaiser Family Foundation. Accessed November 21, 2022. https://www.kff.org/racial-equity-and-health-policy/issue-brief/what-are-the-implications-of-the-overturning-of-roe-v-wade-for-racial-disparities/.

14. Donohue III, John, and Steven Levitt. 2020. "The Impact of Abortion on Crime Over the Last Two Decades." *American Law and Economics Review.* Accessed November 28, 2022. https://law.stanford.edu/publications/the-impact-of-legalized-abortion-on-crime-over-the-last-two-decades/.

15. Pew Research Center. 2022. "Majority of Public Disapproves of Supreme Court's Decision to Overturn Roe v Wade." Accessed November 28, 2022. https://www.pewresearch.org/politics/2022/07/06/majority-of-public-disapproves-of-supreme-courts-decision-to-overturn-roe-v-wade/.

CHAPTER 3

1. Stevens, Rosemary. 1989. *In Sickness and in Wealth*. New York: Basic Books. p. 259.

2. Kissel, Chris. 2023. "Largest Health Insurance Companies." *Forbes.* Accessed January 3, 2023. https://www.forbes.com/advisor/health-insurance/largest-health-insurance-companies/.

3. Jensen, Gail, et al. 1997. "The New Dominance of Managed Care: Insurance Trends in the 1990s." *Health Affairs.* Accessed November 17, 2022. https://www.healthaffairs.org/doi/abs/10.1377/hlthaff.16.1.125?journalCode=hlthaff.

4. O'Leary, Leif. 2021. "Are Employer-Sponsored Health Plans on Their Way Out?" *Harvard Business Review*. Accessed November 18, 2022. https://hbr.org/2021 /05/are-employer-sponsored-health-plans-on-their-way-out.

5. Kaiser Family Foundation. 2022. "2022 Employer Health Benefits Survey." Accessed November 16, 2022. https://www.kff.org/health-costs/report/2022 -employer-health-benefits-survey/.

6. Taylor, Erin Audrey, et al. 2016. *Consumer Decision Making in the Health Care Marketplace*. Santa Monica, CA: Rand Corporation. Accessed November 16, 2022. https://www.rand.org/content/dam/rand/pubs/research_reports/RR1500/RR1567/ RAND_RR1567.pdf.

7. Reinhardt, Uwe. 2019. *Priced Out: The Economic and Ethical Costs of American Health Care*. Princeton, NJ: Princeton University Press.

8. Brownlee, Shannon. 2007. *Overtreated: Why Too Much Medicine Is Making Us Sicker and Poorer*. New York: Bloomsbury USA.

9. "Marketplace Insurers Denied Nearly 1 in 5 In-Network Claims in 2020, Though It's Often Not Clear Why." 2022. Kaiser Family Foundation. Accessed November 2, 2022.

10. Gray, Bradford. 1986. *Institution of Medicine (US) Committee on Implications of For-Profit Enterprise in Health Care*. Washington, DC: National Academies Press.

11. Minemyer, Paige. 2022. "Which Insurer Was the Most Profitable in Q2? The Answer Won't Surprise You." Fierce Healthcare. Accessed November 1, 2022. https://www.fiercehealth care.com/payers/which-insurer-was-most-profitable-q2-answer-wont-surprise-you.

12. Montague, Alexandra, Katherine Gudiksen, and Jaime King. 2021. "State Action to Oversee Consolidation of Health Care Providers." Milbank Memorial Fund. Accessed November 4, 2022. https://www.milbank.org/publications/state-action-to -oversee-consolidation-of-health-care-providers/.

13. Kazel, Robert. 2004. "Union Seeks to Limit Aetna Execs' Pay." *American Medical News.* Accessed October 28, 2022.

14. White House. 2022. "Fact Sheet: White House Announces over $40 Billion in American Rescue Plan Investments in Our Workforce—With More Coming." Accessed October 28. 2022. https://www.whitehouse.gov/briefing-room/statements -releases/2022/07/12/fact-sheet-white-house-announces-over-40-billion-in-american -rescue-plan-investments-in-our-workforce-with-more-coming/.

15. "1 in 10 Adults Owe Medical Debt, With Millions Owing More than $10,000." 2022. Kaiser Family Foundation. Accessed November 16, 2022. https://www.kff.org /health-costs/press-release/1-in-10-adults-owe-medical-debt-with-millions-owing -more-than-10000/.

16. Schulte, Fred. 2022. "Sick Profit: Investigating Private Equity's Stealthy Take-over of Health Care Across Cities and Specialties." Kaiser Health News. Accessed November 14, 2022. https://khn.org/news/article/private-equity-takeover-health-care -cities-specialties/.

CHAPTER 4

1. Pear, Robert, and Edmund Andrews. 2004. "White House Says Congressional Estimate of New Medicare Costs Was Too Low." *New York Times.* Accessed October 3, 2022. https://www.nytimes.com/2004/02/02/us/white-house-says-congressional -estimate-of-new-medicare-costs-was-too-low.html.

2. Medicare resources.org. n.d. "Find Medicare Plans That Fit Your Needs, catastrophic coverage (Part D)." Accessed October 5, 2022. http://www.medicareresources .org/glossary/catastrophic-coverage/.

3. Hostetter, Martha, and Sarah Klein. 2022. "Taking Stock of Medicare Advantage Risk Adjustment." The Commonwealth Fund. Accessed October 7, 2022. https: //www.commonwealthfund.org/blog/2022/taking-stock-medicare-advantage-risk -adjustment.

4. Freed, Meredith, et al. 2022. "Medicare Advantage in 2022: Enrollment Update and Key Trends." Kaiser Family Foundation. Accessed October 7, 2022. https: //www.kff.org/medicare/issue-brief/medicare-advantage-in-2022-enrollment-update -and-key-trends/.

5. Abelson, Reed, and Margot Sanger-Katz. 2022. "'The Case Monster Was Insatiable': How Insurers Exploited Medicare for Billions." *New York Times.* Accessed October 8, 2022. http://www.nytimes.com/2022/10/08/upshot/medicare-advantage -fraud-allegations.html.

6. Frank, Richard, and Conrad Milhaupt. 2022. "Profits, Medical Loss-ratios, and the Ownership Structure of Medicare Advantage Plans." *USC-Brookings Schaeffer on Health Policy.* Accessed October 6, 2022. https://www.brookings.edu/blog/ usc-brookings-schaeffer-on-health-policy/2022/07/13/profits-medical-loss-ratios-and -the-ownership-structure-of-medicare-advantage-plans/

7. Jacobson, Gretchen, and David Blumenthal. 2022. "Medicare Advantage Enrollment Growth: Implications for the US Health Care System." *Journal of the American Medical Association.* Accessed October 6, 2022. doi:10.1001/jama.2022.8288.

8. Ethridge, Lynn, and Judith Moore. 2003. "A New Medicaid Program," *Health Affairs.* Accessed October 18, 2022. http://content.healthaffairs.org/content/early /2003/08/27/hlthaff.w3.426/suppl/DC1.

9. Guth, Madeline, and MaryBeth Musumeci. 2022. "An Overview of Medicaid Work Requirements: What Happened Under Trump and Biden Administrations?" Kaiser Family Foundation. Accessed October 18, 2022. https://www.kff.org/medicaid /issue-brief/an-overview-of-medicaid-work-requirements-what-happened-under-the -trump-and-biden-administrations/

10. "Raising the Age of Medicare Eligibility: A Fresh Look Following Implementation of Health Reform." 2011. Henry J. Kaiser Family Foundation Program on Medicare Policy, publication number 8169. Accessed October 21, 2022. http://www .kff.org/Medicare/upload/8169.pdf.

CHAPTER 5

1. Imber, Gerald. 2011. *Genius on the Edge: The Bizarre Double Life of William Stewart Halsted.* New York: Kaplan Publishing.

2. Willis, Antono, et al. 2021. "The State of Primary Care in the United States: A Chartbook of Facts and Statistics." Robert Graham Center. www.grapham-center.org; IBM-Watson Health (IBM). www.ibm.com/watson-health; The American Board of Family Medicine (ABFM)& affiliated Center for Professionalism &Value in Health Care (CPV) http://professionalismandvalue.org. Accessed December 5, 2022.

3. Bitten, Asaf. 2022. "The Case for Investing in Primary Care." The Commonwealth Fund, The Dose (podcast). Accessed December 2, 2022. https://www .commonwealthfund.org/publications/podcast/2022/mar/case-investing-primary -care.

4. Schulte, Fred. 2022. "Sick Profit: Investigating Private Equity's Stealthy Takeover of Health Care Across Cities and Specialties." Kaiser Health News. Accessed Nov. 14, 2022. https://khn.org/news/article/private-equity-takeover-health-care-cities -specialties/.

5. American Medical Association. 2023. "Medicare Physician Payment Schedule." Accessed January 9, 2023. https://www.ama-assn.org/practice-management/medicare -medicaid/medicare-physician-payment-schedule.

6. Sharma, Rahul, and Lynn Carroll. 2022. "How Physicians Can Untangle the Web of Relationships for Value-based Success." *Medical Economics.* Accessed December 5, 2022. https://www.medicaleconomics.com/view/how-physicians-can-untangle-the -web-of-relationships-essential-for-value-based-care-success.

7. Shanafelt, Tait, et al. 2022. "Changes in Burnout and Satisfaction With Work-Life Integration in Physicians During First 2 Years of Covid-19 Pandemic." *Mayo Clinic Proceedings.* Accessed December 6, 2022. https://www.mayoclinicproceedings.org/ article/S0025-6196(22)00515-8/fulltext.

8. Reinhart, Eric. 2023. "Doctors Aren't Burned Out from Overwork. We're Demoralized by Our Health System." *New York Times.* Accessed February 8, 2023. https://www.nytimes.com/2023/02/05/opinion/doctors-universal-health-care.html.

9. Salmon, J. Warren, and Stephen Thompson. 2021. *The Corporatization of American Health Care: The Rise of Corporate Hegemony and Loss of Professional Autonomy.* New York: Springer Publishing.

10. Sage, William, Richard Boothman, and Thomas Gallagher. 2020. "Another Medical Malpractice Crisis?" *Journal of the American Medical Association* 324(14): 1395–96. Accessed December 6, 2022. https://jamanetwork.com/journals/jama/ fullarticle/2770929.

CHAPTER 6

1. "Hospital Beds (per 1,000 people)." World Bank, based on World Health Organization figures, 1960–2019. n.d. Accessed September 16, 2022. https://data.worldbank .org/indicator/SH.MED.BEDS.ZS.

2. Corwin, E. H. L. 1946. *The American Hospital*. New York: Commonwealth Fund.

3. "Hospital Service in the United States." *Journal of the American Medical Association* 90 (April 3, 1928): 1009. Accessed September 19, 2022. https://jamanetwork .com/journals/jama/article-abstract/255163.

4. Galewitz, Phil. 2022. "Hospitals Divert Primary Care Patients to Health Center 'Look-Alikes' to Boost Finances." Kaiser Health News. Accessed September 9, 2022. https://khn.org/news/article/hospitals-divert-primary-care-patients-health-center-look -alikes/.

5. CDC Fact Sheet. n.d. "Hospital Utilization (in nonfederal short-stay hospitals)." Accessed September 16, 2022. http://cdc.gov/nchs/fastats/hospital.htm.

6. Sebelius, Kathleen. 2013. "The Affordable Care Act at Three: Paying for Quality Saves Health Care Dollars," *Health Affairs*. Accessed September 16, 2022. https: //www.healthaffairs.org/do/10.1377/forefront.20130320.029408.

7. Manjoua, Youssra, and Kevin Bozic. 2012. "Brief History of Quality Movement in US Healthcare." *Current Reviews of Musculoskeletal Medicine*, 5(4): 265–73. Accessed September 14, 2022.

8. Schwartz, Karyn, et al. 2020. "What We Know About Provider Consolidation." Kaiser Family Foundation. Accessed September 20, 2022. https://www.kff.org/health -costs/issue-brief/what-we-know-about-provider-consolidation/.

9. US Department of Justice. 2003. "Largest Health Care Fraud Case in U.S. History Settled HCA Investigation Nets Record Total of $1.7 Billion." Accessed September 19, 2022.

10. US Department of Justice. 2006. "Tenet Healthcare Corporation to Pay U.S. More Than $900 Million to Resolve False Claims Act Allegations." Accessed September 19, 2022.

11. Mahar, Maggie. 2006. *Money-Driven Medicine: The Real Reason Health Care Costs So Much.* New York: HarperCollins.

12. Farmer, Blake. 2022. "Hospital Giant HCA Fends Off Accusations of Questionable Inpatient Admissions," Nashville Public Radio. Accessed Nov. 4, 2022. https:// khn.org/news/article/hca-hospitals-admissions-accusations/.

13. Malone, Tyler, et al. 2021. "The Economic Effect of Rural Hospital Closures," *Health Services Research*, 57(3): 614–23. Accessed September 26, 2022. https:// onlinelibrary.wiley.com/doi/full/10.1111/1475–6773.13965.

14. Offodile, Anaeze, et al. 2021. "Private Equity Investments in Health Care: An Overview of Hospital and Health System Leveraged Buyouts, 2003–17." *Health Affairs*, 5(2021): 719–26. Accessed November 14, 2022; Lee, Chris. 2022. "KFF's Kaiser Health News Investigates Private Equity's Stealth Takeover of Health Care in the United States." Kaiser Family Foundation. Accessed November 14, 2022. https: //www.kff.org/health-costs/press-release/kffs-kaiser-health-news-investigates-private -equitys-stealth-takeover-of-health-care-in-the-united-states/.

15. Letchuman, Sunjay, et al. 2022. "Revise the IRS's Nonprofit Hospital Community Benefit Reporting Standard." *Health Affairs* Forefront. Accessed November 3, 2022. https://www.healthaffairs.org/do/10.1377/forefront.20220413.829370.

16. Levinson, Zachery, Scott Hulver, and Tricia Neuman. 2022. "Hospital Charity Care: How It Works and Why It Matters." Kaiser Family Foundation. Accessed

November 3, 2022. https://www.kff.org/health-costs/issue-brief/hospital-charity-care
-how-it-works-and-why-it-matters/.

17. "How Nonprofit Hospitals Put Profits Over Patients." 2023. *New York Times* podcast. Accessed January 25, 2023. https://www.nytimes.com/2023/01/25/podcasts/the-daily/nonprofit-hospitals-investigation.html.

18. Silver-Greenberg, Jessica, and Katie Thomas. 2022. "They Were Entitled to Free Care. Hospitals Hounded Them to Pay." *New York Times*. Accessed November 24, 2022. https://www.nytimes.com/2022/09/24/business/nonprofit-hospitals-poor-patients.html.

19. National Nurses United. 2020. "New Study—Hospitals Hike Charges by Up to 18 Times Cost." Press Release. Accessed November 24, 2022. https://www.nationalnursesunited.org/press/new-study-hospitals-hike-charges-18-times-cost/.

20. Horwitz, Jill, and Austin Nichols. 2022. "Hospital Service Offerings Still Differ Substantially By Ownership Type." *Health Affairs*, 41(3): 331–40. Accessed November 24, 2022. https://www.healthaffairs.org/doi/abs/10.1377/hlthaff.2021.01115.

21. Jeurissen, Patrick, et al. 2021 "For-Profit Hospitals Have Thrived Because of Generous Public Reimbursement Schemes, Not Greater Efficiency: A Multi-Country Case Study." *International Journal of Health Services*, 51(1): 167–89. Accessed November 24, 2022. https://doi.org/10.1177/0020731420966976.

22. Chan, David, David Card, and Lowell Taylor. 2021. "Is There a VA Advantage? Evidence from Dually Eligible Veterans." Paper. Accessed November 24, 2022. (March) https://www.bu.edu/econ/files/2021/04/paper.pdf.

23. Kofman, Ava. 2022. "Endgame: How the Visionary Hospice Movement Became a For-Profit Hustle." ProPublica. Accessed November 28, 2022. https://www.propublica.org/article/hospice-healthcare-aseracare-medicare.

24. Adler, Loren, et al. 2023. "Ground Ambulance Billing Prices Differ by Ownership Structure." *Health Affairs*. Accessed January 18, 2023. https://www.healthaffairs.org/doi/10.1377/hlthaff.2022.00738.

25. Gee, Emily. 2019. "The High Price of Hospital Care." Center for American Progress. Accessed November 6, 2022. https://www.americanprogress.org/article/high-price-hospital-care/.

26. Weismann, Dan. 2023. "Can They Freaking Do That?!?! (2023 edition)." An Arm and A Leg Podcast, Kaiser Health News. Accessed February 6, 2023. https://khn.org/news/podcast/an-arm-and-a-leg-can-they-freaking-do-that-2023-update/.

CHAPTER 7

1. McCarthy, Justin. 2019. "Big Pharma Sinks to the Bottom of U.S. Industry Ratings." *Gallup*. Accessed December 13, 2022. https://news.gallup.com/poll/266060/big-pharma-sinks-bottom-industry-rankings.aspx.

2. Hamel, Liz, et al. 2022. "Public Opinion on Prescription Drugs and Their Prices." Kaiser Family Foundation. Accessed October 20, 2022. https://www.kff.org/health-costs/poll-finding/public-opinion-on-prescription-drugs-and-their-prices/.

3. Moore, Thomas, et al. 2020. "Variation in the Estimated Costs of Pivotal Clinical Trials Supporting the US Approval of New Therapeutic Agents, 2015–2017: A Cross-sectional Study." *British Medical Journal*, published online. Accessed December 13, 2022. https://pubmed.ncbi.nlm.nih.gov/32532786/.

4. ClinicalTrials.gov. n.d. "Trends, Charts, and Maps." Accessed December 15, 2022. https://clinicaltrials.gov/ct2/resources/trends.

5. Pradhan, Rachana. 2022. "The Business of Clinical Trials Is Booming. Private Equity Has Taken Notice." Kaiser Health News. Accessed December 2, 2022. https://khn.org/news/article/business-clinical-trials-private-equity.

6. Salib, Veronica. n.d. "How Pharmaceutical Patents Contribute to Increased Drug Costs." *PharmanewsIntelligencer*. Accessed Dec. 2, 2022. https://pharmanewsintel.com/features/how-pharmaceutical-patents-contribute-to-increased-drug-costs/.

7. Jewett, Christina. 2022. "FDA's Drug Fees Fuel Concerns Over Influence." *New York Times*. Accessed December 15, 2022. https://www.nytimes.com/2022/09/15/health/fda-drug-industry-fees.html.

8. Abrams Kaplan, Deborah. 2021. "Generic Drug Price Tags: Too High. And Too Low. Competition Can Help Create an In-Between." *Managed Healthcare Executive*. Accessed December 14, 2022. https://www.managedhealthcareexecutive.com/view/generic-drug-price-tags-too-high-and-too-low-competition-can-help-create-an-in-between-/.

9. Fox, Erin. 2017. "How Pharma Companies Game the System to Keep Drugs Expensive." *Harvard Business Review*. Accessed December 12. 2022. https://hbr.org/2017/04/how-pharma-companies-game-the-system-to-keep-drugs-expensive.

10. Miller, Kathleen, Lewis Fermaglich, and Janet Maynard. 2021. "Using Four Decades of FDA Orphan Designations to Describe Trends in Rare Disease Drug Development: Substantial Growth Seen in Development of Drugs for Rare Oncologic, Neurologic, and Pediatric-onset Diseases." *Orphanet Journal of Rare Diseases*. Accessed December 12, 2022. https://doi.org/10.1186/s13023-021-01901-6.

11. Seeley, Elizabeth. 2022. "The Impact of Pharmaceutical Wholesalers on U.S. Drug Spending." Commonwealth Fund, Issue Briefs. Accessed December 12, 2022. https://www.commonwealthfund.org/publications/issue-briefs/2022/jul/impact-pharmaceutical-wholesalers-drug-spending/.

12. Sood, Neeraj, and Karen Van Nuys, 2022. "The Cantwell-Grassley PBM Bill Is Much Needed But More Can Be Done." *Health Affairs*. Accessed December 19, 2022.

13. Allen, Arthur. 2022. "Pharma-Funded FDA Gets Drugs Out Faster, But Some Work Only 'Marginally' and Most Are Pricey." Kaiser Health News. Accessed September 30, 2022. https://khn.org/news/article/pharma-fda-drugs-accelerated-approval-marginally-effective-expensive/.

14. Fein, Adam. 2022. "The Top U.S. Pharmacies of 2021: Market Share and Revenues of the Biggest Companies." *Drug Channels.* Accessed Dec. 12, 2022. https://www.drugchannels.net/2022/03/the-top-15-us-pharmacies-of-2021-market.html.

15. Allen, Arthur. 2022. "How Pfizer Won the Pandemic, Reaping Outsize Profits and Influence." Kaiser Health News. Accessed December 12, 2022. https://khn.org/news/article/pfizer-pandemic-vaccine-market-paxlovid-outsize-profit-influence/.

16. Clark, Bobby, and Jeff Callis. 2022. "Public Good vs. Private Gain: The Role of Public-Private Partnerships in Drug Innovations and Pricing." Commonwealth Fund, Blog. Accessed December 14, 2022. https://www.commonwealthfund.org/blog /2022/public-good-vs-private-gain-role-public-private-partnerships-drug-innovation -and-pricing.

17. Rajkumar, S. Vincent. 2020. "The High Cost of Prescription Drugs: Causes and Solutions." *Blood Cancer Journal* 10 (71). Accessed December 6, 2022. https://doi .org/10.1038/s41408-020-0338-x.

18. Feldman, Robin. 2021. "Drug Companies Keep Merging. Why That's Bad for Consumers and Innovation." *Washington Post.* Accessed December 6, 2022. https:// www.washingtonpost.com/outlook/2021/04/06/drug-companies-keep-merging-why -thats-bad-consumers-innovation/.

19. Buntz, Brian. 2020. "GSK, Pfizer and J&J Among the Most-fined Drug Companies." *Pharmaceutical Processing World.* Accessed December 7, 2022. https:// www.pharmaceuticalprocessingworld.com/gsk-pfizer-and-jj-among-the-most-fined -drug-companies-according-to-study/.

CHAPTER 8

1. Statista. "2022 Percentage of Respondents World Wide Who Were Satisfied With Their Nations's Health System as of 2019 by Country." Accessed January 9, 2023. https://www.statista.com/statistics/1109036/satisfaction-health-system-worldwide-by -country/.

2. Anderson, Odin. 1972. *Health Care: Can There Be Equity? The United States, Sweden, and England.* New York: Wiley-Interscience.

3. Jolley, Rachael, ed. 2013. "State of the Nation: Where Is Bittersweet Britain Heading?" *British Future.* Accessed January 9, 2023. https://www.britishfuture.org/ wp-content/uploads/2020/09/State-of-the-Nation-2013.pdf.

4. Cheng, Tsung-Mei. 2010. "Understanding the 'Swiss Watch' Function of Switzerland's Health System." *Health Affairs.* Accessed January 9, 2023. https://www .healthaffairs.org/doi/abs/10.1377/hlthaff.2010.0698.

5. Grossman, David, and Barbara Choucair. 2019. "Violence and the U.S. Health Care Sector: Burden and Response." *Health Affairs*. Accessed February 22, 2023. https://www.healthaffairs.org/doi/10.1377/hlthaff.2019.00642.

6. Durand-Zaleski, Isabelle. 2020. "International Health Care System Profiles." The Commonwealth Fund. Accessed January 6, 2023. https://www.commonwealthfund .org/international-health-policy-center/countries/france.

Center for Restorative Breast Surgery. 2021. "Health Care in France: Is This the World's Best Health Care?" Accessed January 6, 2023. https://www.breastcenter.com /2021/11/07/health care-in-france-is-this-the-worlds-best-health care-system/.

7. Schneider, Eric, et al. 2020. "Mirror, Mirror 2021: Reflecting Poorly," (Aug. 4, 2020) The Commonwealth Fund. Accessed Nov. 18, 2022. https://www .commonwealthfund.org/publications/fund-reports/2021/aug/mirror-mirror-2021 -reflecting-poorly.

European Observatory on Health Systems and Policies. 2022. "Book Launch—Health Systems Performance Assessment: A Framework for Policy Analysis." U-Tube video. Accessed November 18, 2022. https://www.youtube.com/watch?v=02xIz5kEtTo

8. OECDiLibrary. 2019. "Health at a Glance 2019: OECD Indicators." Avoidable Mortality (Preventable and Treatable). Accessed November 17, 2022. https://www.oecd-ilibrary.org/sites/3b4fdbf2-en/index.html?itemId=/content/component/3b4fdbf2-en.

CHAPTER 9

1. World Health Organization. 2017. "Determinants of Health." Accessed October 7, 2022. https://www.who.int/news-room/questions-and-answers/item/determinants-of-health.

2. World Health Organization. n.d. "Social Determinants of Health." Accessed October 7, 2022. https://www.who.int/health-topics/social-determinants-of-health#tab=tab_1.

3. World Health Organization. "Determinants of Health."

4. Stiglitz, Joseph. 2018. "The American Economy Is Rigged." *Scientific American*. Accessed October 12, 2022. https://www.scientificamerican.com/article/the-american-economy-is-rigged/.

5. Siripurapu, Anshu. Council on Foreign Relations. 2022. "The US Inequality Debate." Accessed October 14, 2022. https://www.cfr.org/backgrounder/us-inequality-debate.

6. Marmot, M.G., et al. 1991. "Health Inequalities among British Civil Servants: The Whitehall II Study." *The Lancet*. Accessed October 17, 2022. https://www.thelancet.com/journals/lancet/article/PII0140-6736(91)93068-K/fulltext.

7. Kawachi, Ichiro, Bruce Kennedy, and Richard Wilkinson (eds.). 1991. *The Social Population Health Reader: Income Inequality and Health*. New York: New Press.

8. Zajacova, Anna, and Elizabeth Lawrence. 2019. "The Relationship between Education and Health: Reducing Disparities through a Contextual Approach." *Annual Review of Public Health*. Accessed December 20, 2022. https://www.annualreviews.org/doi/abs/10.1146/annurev-publhealth-031816-044628.

9. Siripurapu. "The US Inequality Debate."

10. Weston, Liz. 2014. "OECD: The U.S. Has Fallen Behind Other Countries in College Completion," Reuters. Accessed June 6, 2023. https://www.businessinsider.com/r-us-falls-behind-in-college-competition-oecd-2014-9#:~:text=In%201995%2C%20the%20United%20States,of%20college%20graduates%2C%20Schleicher%20said.

11. Desilver, Drew. 2020. "U.S. Students' Academic Achievement Still Lags Behind That of Their Peers in Many Other Countries," PEW Research Center. Accessed Jan. 25, 2023. https://www.pewresearch.org/short-reads/2017/02/15/u-s-students-internationally-math-science/.

12. American Public Health Association. 2017. "Reducing Income Inequality to Advance Health." APHA Policy Statement 9204: Labor Unions and Health. Policy. Accessed December 20, 2022. https://www.apha.org/policies-and-advocacy/public -health-policy-statements/policy-database/2018/01/18/reducing-income-inequality-to -advance-health.

13. Ibid.

14. Case, Ann, and Angus Deaton. 2020. *Deaths of Despair and the Future of Capitalism*. Princeton, NJ: Princeton University Press.

15. APHA Policy Statement #20179.

16. American Public Health Association. 2017. "Reducing Income Inequality to Advance Health. Policy #20179 Accessed December 20, 2022. https://www.apha.org /policies-and-advocacy/public-health-policy-statements/policy-database/2018/01/18/ reducing-income-inequality-to-advance-health.

17. Bollyky, T. J., et al. 2022. "Pandemic Preparedness and Covid-19: An Exploratory Analysis of Infection and Fatality Rates, and Contextual Factors Associated with Preparedness in 177 Countries, from Jan. 1, 2020, to Sept. 30, 2021." *Lancet.* Accessed Dec. 20, 2022. doi.org/10.1016/S0140-6736(22)00172-6.

18. Cunningham, Timothy, et al. 2017. "Morbidity and Mortality Weekly Report (MMWR)." Centers for Disease Control and Prevention. Accessed December 20, 2022. https://www.cdc.gov/mmwr/volumes/66/wr/mm6617e1.htm.

19. Ibid.

20. "Racism-induced Stress Linked with High Black Infant Mortality Rates." 2017. Harvard T. H. Chan School of Public Health, News. Accessed January 17, 2023. hhttps://www.hsph.harvard.edu/news/hsph-in-the-news/racism-induced-stress-black -infant-mortality/.

21. Orminski, Emily. 2021. "Your Zip Code Is More Important Than Your Genetic Code." National Community Reinvestment Coalition. Accessed December 16, 2022. https://ncrc.org/your-zip-code-is-more-important-than-your-genetic-code/.

22. Marmot, Michael. 2005. *The Status Syndrome: How Social Standing Affects Our Health and Longevity.* New York: MacMillan.

23. Amenabar, Teddy. 2023. "Want to Be Healthier? Hang Out With Your Friends." *Washington Post.* Accessed January 9, 2023. https://www.washingtonpost.com/ wellness/2023/01/09/how-to-adult-friends-relationships.

24. McKinlay, John. 2019. "A Case for Refocusing Upstream: The Political Economy of Illness." IAPHA Occasional Classics. Accessed October 4, 2022. https://iaphs .org/wp-content/uploads/2019/11/IAPHS-McKinlay-Article.pdf.

25. Stiglitz. "The American Economy Is Rigged."

26. Menasce Horowitz, Juliana, Ruth Igielnik, and Rakesh Kochhar. 2020. "More Americans Say There Is Too Much Economic Inequality in the U.S., But Fewer than Half Call It a Top Priority." Pew Research Center. Accessed December 16, 2022. https://www.pewresearch.org/social-trends/2020/01/09/most-americans-say-there-is -too-much-economic-inequality-in-the-u-s-but-fewer-than-half-call-it-a-top-priority.

27. "Public Trust in Government, 1958–2022." Pew Research Center. 2022. Accessed December 16, 2022. https://www.pewresearch.org/politics/2022/06/06/ public-trust-in-government-1958-2022/.

28. Ingraham, Christopher. 2020. "U.N. Warns That Runaway Inequality Is Destabilizing the World's Democracies." *Washington Post.* Accessed December 20, 2022. https://www.washingtonpost.com/business/2020/02/11/income-inequality-un -destabilizing/.

Index

AbbVie, 102
Aetna, 39
Accountable Care Organization (ACO), 50, 69
Affordable Care Act (ACA), vii, 1, 23, 30–41, 47–48, 52–53, 88, 92, 108
Agency for Healthcare Research and Quality (AHRQ), 12, 89
Agency for Toxic Substance and Diseases Registry (ATSDR), 12
allopaths, 60–61, 66
Alternative Payment Models (APMs), 69
American Association of Physicians Assistants (AAPA), 76
American College of Physicians (ACP), 82
American College of Surgeons (ACS), 82
American Hospital Association (AHA), 68, 82, 90
American Journal of Public Health, 15
American Medical Association (AMA), 12, 25, 27, 64, 66–68, 70–71, 83
American Nurses Association (ANA), 74
American Public Health Association (APHA), vii, 15, 134, 136

American Rescue Plan Act (ARPA), 40, 53
Association of American Medical Colleges (AAMC), 64–65
Anthem, 26

Blue Cross, 23–26, 85
Blue Cross-Blue Shield (BC-BS), 25, 27, 32, 68
Bayh-Dole Act, 106
Bureau of Labor Statistics (BLS), 59

Canadian healthcare system, 112–16
capitation, 25, 118
Centene, 39
Centers for Disease Control and Prevention (CDC), 11, 14, 59
Centers for Medicare and Medicaid Services (CMS), 48–49, 59, 67–68, 89
Chargemaster, 94
Childrens Health Insurance Program (CHIP), 44, 55–56
Cigna, 104
Consolidated Omnibus Budget Reconciliation Act (COBRA), 35
consumer-driver healthcare, 27, 30, 34, 39, 97